About the Series

IDEAS IN PROGRESS is a commercially published series of working papers dealing with alternatives to industrial society. It is our belief that the ills and profound frustrations which have overtaken man are not merely due to industrial civilization's inadequate planning and faulty execution, but are caused by fundamental errors in our basic thinking about goals. This series is designed to question and rethink the underlying concepts of many of our institutions and to propose alternatives. Unless this is done soon society will undoubtedly create even greater injustices and inequalities than at present. It is to correct this trend that authors are invited to submit short texts of work in progress of interest not only to their colleagues but also to the general public. The series fosters direct contact between the author and the reader. It provides the author with the opportunity to give wide circulation to his draft while he is still developing an idea. It offers the reader an opportunity to participate critically in shaping this idea before it has taken on a definitive form.

Readers are invited to write directly to the authors of the present volume at the following address:
Professors Manu L. Kothari and Lopa A. Mehta, Seth G. S. Medical College, Parel, Bombay, 400012 INDIA.

THE PUBLISHERS

Ideas in Progress

CANCER

Myths and Realities
of Cause and Cure

Manu L. Kothari (MBBS, MS, MSC [MED])
Lopa A. Mehta (MBBS, MS)

LONDON
MARION BOYARS
BOSTON

Published simultaneously in Great Britain and the United States in
1979
by Marion Boyars Ltd.
18 Brewer Street, London W1R 4AS.
and Marion Boyars Inc.
99 Main Street, Salem, New Hampshire 03079

Australian distribution by Thomas C. Lothian
4-12 Tattersalls Lane, Melbourne, Victoria 3000.

Published in Canada by Burns & MacEachern Ltd.
Suite 3, Railside Road, Don Mills, Ontario M3A 1A6

ISBN 0 7145 2665 7 cased edition
ISBN 0 7145 2666 5 paper edition

Filmset in Monophoto Baskerville 169
by A. Brown & Sons Ltd., Hull, England.

CONTENTS

J UST as key decisions on energy, on atomic generators, on fast breeders, on the storage of waste must be controlled by enlightened voters, so the basic policies on cancer research and cancer treatment facilities must be brought under the political surveillance of the general public.

This is the first book that puts the layman into the position to *use* expert advice rather than *be used* by the expert.

Ivan Illich
Cuernavaca, Mexico

T HIS book preaches revolution within the politics of health. The diminishing returns of contemporary medicine is a theme which has become familiar; here, however we find it extended into that territory most jealously guarded by the proponents of high technology and the keepers of the charitable purse: cancer. The medical management of cancer is the paradigm of the commodity approach to health, based on the doctrine of specific etiology (a specific cause for every disease) and the mechanistic therapeutics of body as automobile. In presenting their natural theory of cancer Kothari and Metha provide a challenge, rooted in the evidence of their professions, which the world-wide cancer industry will find it difficult to ignore. They also provide a hope that the sacrifice encouraged by the radical critics of Western health care in moving away from a tradition of professional dominance may be nothing like as great as has hitherto been feared.

Alex Scott-Samuel
Community physician
Liverpool, England

PREFACE

CANCER is a subject of fascination and fear, in minds medical and lay. This need no longer be. Cancer, when viewed in a gestalt biological perspective, loses its air of malignancy and mystery and becomes understandable. Einstein once remarked that the most incomprehensible thing about the world is that it is comprehensible. The same could be said of cancer – comprehensible as much by the layman as by the learned.

As the title suggests, the thrust of this book is iconoclastic. It explodes the myths about cancer, and exposes the realities – a presentation based on scientific references and woven into an integrated thesis. The cause and the cure of cancer cannot be known – they are just not there. Depressing? Hardly. The facts that inexorably lead to the foregoing conclusions provide us all with the logical insight not to fear the occurrence of cancer on the one hand and to be able to live with it, on the other.

In June 1973, we presented our views – the cancer realistic approach – as *The Nature of Cancer*, Volume one. It received respectful criticism when reviewed in international journals. The passage of 5 years and the oceanic work and literature on cancer have not necessitated any significant change in the contents of the book.

We met Ivan Illich when he visited Bombay in February 1978. He inspired us to write a brief, non-technical account of our views for a wider, non-medical readership, and hence this book. The citation of references all along will, it is hoped, aid both the reader as well as the text – the reader to satisfy his curiosity, and the text to withstand any scientific scrutiny.

We are thankful to Ivan Illich for his help and encouragement. Professor Sunil Pandya, Professor Surendra Bhatnagar, Dr. Jyoti Kothari and Rajesh Parikh have critically read the manuscript to help us arrange the ideas in a logical sequence.

It has been a pleasure to work with Marion Boyars. She has been of inestimable help in editing and simplifying the text. Her letters to us, while effectively bridging the distance between London and Bombay, have significantly enhanced the purpose of the book.

Manu Kothari
Lopa Mehta

ONE

THE MYTHS OF CANCER

THE dictionary[1] defines *myth* as a belief given uncritical acceptance by the members of a group especially in support of existing or traditional practices and institutions. The mythology of cancer includes such 'facts' as, that cancer is *caused* by an agent, (and hence can be *prevented* by ridding humanity of that agent), that it can be *diagnosed* at a stage when a preemptive strike at it would assure a *cure*, and that these are the essentials that need bother us about the *nature* of cancer. Never in the history of mankind has so much untruth been told so often by so few to so many, and that these are the essentials that need bother us about the mythology of cancer can be summed up as *ignorance*, matched by *overclaiming*, *overdoing* and *overpromising*.

Our ignorance starts with the apparently simple problem of defining cancer. Virchow[2], the father of cellular pathology, remarked in the last century that no man, even under torture, could define cancer. The passage of the century has made no change in the Virchowian conclusion; Foulds[3], the

British cancerologist, recently stated that cancer research will reach 'an outstanding landmark' the day it can define cancer in biological terms.

Such fundamental ignorance explains the state of cancerology today – 'scientifically bankrupt, therapeutically ineffective, and wasteful.' This candour, by Nobel prize-winner Watson[4] of *Double Helix* fame, was worded differently by another Nobel prize-winner, Burnet[5], when he stated that if there could be 'a comprehensive and unbiased survey of cancer research,' the surveyor would end up with a devastating sense of futility – the end-result of the hundreds of thousands of man-years of work on the various aspects of cancer has been 'precisely nil.' Whither cancerology?

Despite doctors' exhortations to diagnose early, remember[6, 7, 8] the number of eminent cancerologists who have fallen victim to the disease they were trying to conquer. One of the earliest was Armand Trousseau, the great clinician of *Hôtel Dieu de Paris* who recognized migrating thrombophlebitis – Trousseau's syndrome, described by him – as the first sign of his own advanced abdominal cancer. William Mayo, co-founder of the famous Mayo Clinic, who wrote some classic papers on the surgery of stomach cancer, accidentally felt his own advanced cancer, as did Sir D. P. D. Wilkie of England, another notable name in surgery. James Ewing, the famous pathologist and research director of the Memorial Hospital, New York, died of bladder cancer. Close by us is the Tata Memorial Centre, an exclusive cancer hospital and research centre. Two surgeons from there, Ernest Borges and Sorab Mehta had their cancers diagnosed 'too late.' Leslie Foulds, of the Imperial Research Fund and author of the two volume work *Neoplastic Development*, died of a colonic cancer that was very advanced when first diagnosed. Other names include Frank Horsfall, the director of the Sloan-Kettering Institute who died of pancreatic cancer, and David Karnofsky, chief of SKI's chemotherapy section, who died of lung cancer. Dorn, one of the most notable names in cancer epidemiology, died of kidney cancer. Shakespeare aptly aphorized that 'By medicine life may be prolong'd, yet death will seize the doctor too.'

By treatment life may be eased, yet cancer can kill the cancerologist too. Solzhenitsyn[9] has portrayed this touchingly in *Cancer Ward*. Ludmila Afanasyevna, radiotherapist of the hero Oleg, develops cancer, about which she hopelessly realizes nothing can be done. The understanding by laymen that the most eminent names in the field of cancer can also get cancer and die of it, will go a long way in assuaging the not uncommon 'why me?' or 'why my—?' complex.

Cancer experts overclaim to breed illusions of knowledge of the causes of cancer. Despite the fact that not one cause (including smoking), advanced by them as responsible for the occurrence of a cancer, has ever proved to be the *sine qua non* of that cancer, cancerology continues to hold everything under the sun, including the sun itself, as cancerogenic. The latest to be added to this plethora of cancerogens is the human sperm. The outcome of it all is *cancerophobia*, a disease, aptly described by Ingelfinger[10] the past editor of the prestigious *New England Journal of Medicine* as 'as serious as cancer itself', and morally far more devastating.

Cancerologists overdo – overdiagnose and overtreat – because they refuse to accept the writing on the wall that no cancer can be diagnosed early enough, or can be treated to the point of a cure: the cancer therapist treats what he sees. The illusion of a cure following therapy lies mainly in the patient *not feeling* the presence of cancer and/or the clinician *not being able to detect* it. The classic example is that of acute leukemia where even in 'complete remission' [45, 98, 265] the patient's body has a large number of cancer cells all the time. (See Chapter 6).

13

Hardin Jones[11], from an extensive survey of varied cancers, concluded: 'It is most likely that, in terms of life expectancy, the chance of survival is no better with than without treatment, and there is the possibility that treatment may make the survival time of cancer cases less.'

Jones's 1956 assessment was reinforced in 1975 by Logan[12] of the WHO, who from a global survey of breast cancer summarized that despite all the therapeutic radicalism, the mortality had not declined and had possibly increased. Thomas Dao[13], of the Department of Breast Surgery, Rosewell Park Memorial Institute, Buffalo, put it more explicitly: 'Despite improved surgical techniques, advanced methods in radiotherapies, and widespread use of chemotherapies, breast cancer mortality has not changed in the last 70 years.' This cancer occurs just beneath the skin. Its natural history has been studied for centuries. It is one of the most amenable tumours to self-examination, clinical examination, staging, grading, hormone therapy, and what have you. Breast cancer, as a paradigm, typifies the utter failure of cancerology. When and how should cancerology reveal this truth to the public? Left to cancerologists, it never will.

In a subtle way, cancer societies manipulate minds. When Jane Brody of *The New York Times* joins hands with Arthur Holleb of *The American Cancer Society*, the cancerological optimism takes the shape of a big book reassuringly titled *You Can Fight Cancer and Win.*[14] Written in reporters' journalese, the book is replete with such clichés as 'Know Thine Enemy,' 'Cancer Is Conquerable,' and so on, and appears to be more of an advertising campaign for the cancer hospitals and societies.

The Brody-Holleb venture is a typical example of how people can be taken for a ride. For a more objective and balanced approach it is necessary to consult Hixson's *The Patchwork Mouse*,[8] subtitled the 'Politics and Intrigue in the

Campaign to Conquer Cancer.' Hixson's book exposes the scientific double-think perpetrated at the Sloan-Kettering Institute, under the directorship of Robert Good. The sum and substance of Hixson's book: (a) 'The American public, known to the rest of the world as the originator of fads and fetishes, suffers from time to time with a preoccupation over a single disease. Today that disease is cancer . . .' and (b) 'I have some advice for young researchers in biology. Stay out of cancer research because it's full of money and just about out of science.'

The statement (b) above, made by a scientist to Hixson, reveals the most important aspect of the science of cancerology – that it is a non-science, being essentially a political and a fiscal problem, where, as Hixson[8] found out, the main preoccupation is how to 'ask for more cash.' In *Genes, Dreams and Realities* the politics and funding of the non-science of cancer have been most candidly and most pertinently stated by Burnet. [15] He points out that scientists now-a-days have got used to telling 'white lies' – making announcements to justify public support for their own work, knowing full well that their claims that their work 'will help toward discovering the cause and cure of cancer' have no scientific validity.

Regardless, excessive promises abound. June Goodfield,[16] a Fellow of the Royal Society of Medicine, and author of the reportorial book *The Siege of Cancer*, recently asked Robert Good about the eventual outcome. Good's reply was characteristic: 'Just keep the faith, baby. Give us time.' It has been rightly observed that when science leaves, faith begins.

TWO

CANCER AS A BIOLOGICAL PHENOMENON

R EGARDLESS of all the notoriety accorded to it, cancer presents itself as an integral part of biology – a spontaneous, intrinsic, universal phenomenon found in both plant and animal kingdoms, not excluding insects. 'There is no reason to think that cancer is a disease which has been, as it were, superimposed on life. On the contrary, cancer is certainly an integral factor in the evolutionary process, and has a history as long as the type of life which it affects.'[17] It has even been suggested that life, as we understand it today, emerged from the purposeless, incessantly proliferating cancerous mass called pre-life.[18] Stated below are features of cancer that accord it its rightful place in biology.

Cancer Cell and Normal Cell

1. Every normal cell in the body has the potentiality of turning cancerous by the property of cell differentiation – 'a part of its repertoire.'[19] Cell differentiation is the process by

which a cell irreversibly changes its character to turn into another type of cell. The same process by which an embryonic cell changes into a normal liver cell occurs when a normal liver cell turns into a cancerous one.

The human body is made up of a wide variety of cell types – skin, liver, muscle, retina, etc. Although all the cells of an individual have the same genetic content, they manage to develop, look, and behave differently, as distinct cell types, through the as yet ill-understood process called differentiation [253-255] - generally defined as the creation of new types of cells not present earlier. The formation of a cancer cell, from a normal cell of the body at any age, is once again the creation of a distinct, new cell type – one that looks and behaves differently despite having the same genetic content as all the other normal cells of the body. It is now generally agreed [253] that the formation of a cancer cell involves the same process of differentiation as gives rise to normal cells of the body. No wonder that the seemingly gross malfunctioning by cancer cells – such as the secretion of carcinoembryonic antigen (CEA) [256], or ectopic hormones [257] – is now being understood as mere quantitative variations [256, 257] of normal cell function.

2. There is no consistent single, structural, immunological, or biochemical dividing line between a normal cell and its cancerous counterpart. Thus a cancer cell does not have any feature which is not observed in some normal body cell.

The above points can be rendered more clear by taking, say, leukemic cells as an example: 'Since the leukemic cells originate from transformation (cell differentiation) of normal hematopoietic cells, they retain many of the normal cells' properties, and their proliferative behaviour is in many ways similar.' [315] More specifically: 'Attempts to distinguish normal from leukemic cells biochemically have failed to demonstrate qualitative differences in virtually

17

every instance.'[98] Cytokinetically, both leukemic and normal cells demonstrate 'equivalent cell renewal activity.' [98, 258] Nor can they be differentiated morphologically or immunologically.[98]

3. The difference between a normal cell and a cancer cell lies in their behaviour. A cancer cell, unlike a normal cell which only divides to replace cell loss and maintain the constancy of cell number, divides by its own self-determined rhythm without the body's need. Unlike a normal cell, a cancer cell also migrates from its site of origin and colonizes at distant sites.

Cancer in an Individual

1. Each cancer, human or animal, is, to borrow René Dubos' phrase, *unprecedented, unparalleled, and unrepeatable.* The uniqueness of a cancer lies in its cells as also in the way the cells are arranged and behave. This very uniqueness[3, 15, 155, 156] of every cancer rules out the possibility of having any specific drug or vaccine as curative or preventive against cancer. Writing in *The Lancet* on 'Uniqueness of malignant tumours,' Spriggs and co-workers[239] concluded: 'It is impossible to prove the negative – that identical carcinomas never occur – but the present tests confirm an impression, obtained from thousands of cases, that naturally occurring cancers are extremely diverse even when they carry the same diagnostic label.'

2. The course of a cancer is as unpredictable as that of the individual. Having formed, it may not grow; having grown, it may not dis-ease or trouble; having dis-eased, it may not kill. Many a cancer dies with its owner. *hence it is the cancer, and not the therapy given, that determines the outcome in a human being or an animal.*

3. Cancer in its occurrence exhibits a predictable certainty at the level of a herd, but always remains a matter of chance or probability at an individual level. World over, the overall cancer occurrence is one in five humans.[55] One in five is a matter of certainty; which one, is that of probability. This holds good even in animals[21] specially inbred in laboratories for studying cancer-occurrence generation after generation.

4. Cancer is neither hereditary nor familial. It is its very commonness that makes it occasionally seem so. Willis[20] has generalized that most of the 'cancer families' exemplify only the laws of chance. Scheinfeld's[240] incisive comments on the problem – 'Thus, in grandmother, mother and daughter, where all have breast cancers, each of their cancers may be entirely unrelated to the others. . . . The breast cancers in the three generations of women might be no more related than three cases of stomach trouble, one resulting from over-eating, another from drinking bad liquor, and the third due to stomach ulcers.' – made way back in 1939, has a resounding echo in the 'But so what?' reassurance from Frazer Roberts[241]: 'This is a very common condition.'

5. A cancer is, for the owner, a part of his or her own flesh and blood. It cannot be attacked with impunity without damaging other normal tissues. All anticancer agents treat cancer cells in the same manner as they treat all normal cells. This inseparableness of cancer from normal tissues has rendered cancer radiotherapy 'obsolete'[22] and cancer chemotherapy 'an absolute farce.'[22] In the laboratory cancer chemotherapy produces 100% success because the so-called cancer is a transplanted mass of cells that never belonged to the test animal.[6] In the laboratory and by the bedside, chemotherapy is a 100% failure if the cancer is autochthonous, i.e., the one that arose by itself in the individual.[23]

Cancer in a Herd

1. The type of cancer that occurs is species specific – of the kidneys in frogs, of the nasal sinuses in dogs, of the eyes in Hereford cattle, breasts in bitches, as leukemia in Scottish terriers, and as melanoma of the skin in grey horses.[30, 31]

2. A predominant involvement of a particular organ or system is seen in the different races of man too, as exemplified by the very high incidence of stomach cancer in the Japanese who, as a compensation, have the lowest incidence of leukemia in the whole world.[32] This varying prevalence is not dependent on the environment. It is the racial or the ethnic genetic constitution which governs the type of cancer in a given population. The high incidence of stomach cancer is as much a Japanese feature as are the stub nose and the slit eyes.

   However, the total incidence of cancer, in a herd, is determined by genetic constitution of mankind irrespective of racial and geographic variations. Thus the aggregate incidence of cancer remains the same world over. Smithers[165] has generalized that although the anatomic distribution of cancers in different parts of the world is extremely varied, the overall death-rate from cancers at all sites is remarkably constant for humans the world over.

3. The environmentalistic claim[242, 243] that migrants readily develop a cancer profile typical of the host community, made regardless of the 'manifestly inadequate'[244] data and the many difficulties associated with the study of migrants,[244, 293] fails to find support epidemiologically:[245] Japanese migrants in USA maintain the high rates of stomach cancer typical of Japan, as also the characteristic low rates of breast and cervical cancers, and of leukemias.

Cancer as a Senescent Process

1. Cancer is a manifestation of aging, like hardening of arteries, development of cataract, etc. 'Most spontaneous tumours in animals, as in man, occur in middle-aged or elderly animals.'[20] In children, too, cancer is but a form of senescence. (See Chapter 11).

2. As is typical of biologic processes, cancer in its many facets exhibits gaussian (normal/continuous/bell-shaped) distribution, as may be evinced from, say, the age-incidence of a particular cancer in a human population.[6, 20] This may also be true for its other facets such as growth rate, invasiveness, site of origin, size of cells, etc.[6]

Cancer and Death

1. The fatal bite of the cancerous crab often lies in its spread. The spread of a cancer occurs throughout the length and breadth of the body, but usually manifests itself, apart from the original site of occurrence, at four sites – lung, liver, bones, and brain. No place in the body is, however, exempt from this process. The spread of cancer fools the clinician, frustrates the surgeon, and kills the patient. The *when, where,* and *how much* to spread is determined by the inherent nature of a cancer. Treatment of cancer can precipitate its spread.

2. Cancer apparently serves the natural function[24] of herd mortality, which simply means increasing mortality with increasing age. 'The age-specific mortality rate for cancer increases with age in much the same way that the overall rate does.'[25] To put it simply, the increase in mortality rate with age in cancer is similar to the increase in mortality rate with age in general.

The nature of the link between cancer and death is

debatable as may be realized from the computation that, were cancer eliminated altogether from mankind, it would just add a little more than a year to the human lifespan.[26] Animals would fare no better, in the futuramic *World Without Cancer*.[27]

3. Death is a natural function, not dependent on the presence or absence of a particular disease.[28] It would seem death does what it wants to, and gives the pre-death disease a bad name. Zumoff and co-workers[29] analyzed the mortality statistics for series of patients with diverse diseases – liver cirrhosis, metastatic breast cancer, chronic leukemia, and heart attack. 'It was found that the four diseases analyzed shared an unexpected relationship of mortality rate to duration of disease: the basic mortality rate remained constant during the course of disease; prognosis was neither better nor worse for the patient late in the disease than for the patient early in the disease.' The workers[29] concluded that all the above diseases shared a common alteration of 'the undefined physiological systems' that govern susceptibility to aging and dying.

4. The causes of death in human cancer, Jones[11] surmised, have less to do with the extent of cancer growth than with some other explanation of the metabolic state in cancer. Jones[11] emphasized that 'only a fraction of cancer follow-up suggests that death is due to recurrence of the cancer in an advanced state.' Jones[11] pointed out that the death-rate from intercurrent disease, in cancer, is as great as the rate of death from cancer itself. He speculated that there may be a *general metabolic basis* of cancer as a disease, a phenomenon that may explain why our intense search for cancer cures has been very poorly rewarded. '. . . the population that shows cancer may be already aged from the standpoint of intact metabolic function, so that cancer is only one of the manifestations that occurs in this diseased population'.[11]

Summarizing the biologic features of cancer, one could say that the cancer cell is an altered normal cell; that in an individual, cancer exhibits self-determined uniqueness; that at the level of a herd, while the cancer types vary, the total quantum does not, the world over; that cancer is an evident part of overall vertebrate aging and senescence; and that in relation to death, cancer is NOT the villain of the piece, as portrayed.

Were cancer to have ears and a tongue, it would listen to all our wailings and then apologetically declare its helplessness because of its being rooted in the very thing called life. Thanatologists have, rightly, started preaching from public rostra that death is an inevitable, and an indispensable necessity. Can it not occur to us that this is true for cancer also, and that cancer is not a problem but a solution to the problem of dying? Sir George Pickering,[33] Regius Professor of Medicine at Oxford, summed this up well: 'Aging as a preparation for death is a concept so fundamental that it needs emphasizing before we consider the disease of old age. After all, it is these diseases which kill and make way for the new life. Without them none of us would be living as we are today.' And so it is, with cancer. Cancer will be with us till eternity; let it be.

THREE

CANCER AS A HUMAN PROBLEM

C ANCER, Timothy Foote[34] writes, is a mysterious plague that cries out not for philosophy, but for a palliative. The cataloguing of the biological features of cancer in the earlier chapter cannot ameliorate the hurt feelings and the dis-eased body of a cancer patient. Cancer *is* a human problem, as are other diseases, and death. Haldane,[35] the noted geneticist, who died of a rectal cancer, conceded that 'cancer often kills,' only to add with a chuckle, that 'so do cars and sleeping pills.'

What biological understanding can do for a cancer patient, his near ones and even his doctors, is to help them to see and tackle the issue without fear, incrimination, rushing for needless therapies, or the typical *'j'accuse'* from the doctor to the patient because he 'came too late.' Cancer, so often, does *not* mean a death-sentence, and is compatible with long life. Freud, the father of modern psychiatry, developed cancer of the mouth at the age of 67, and died of something different altogether, at the age of 83.[36] It is not for

24

us to choose the *whether, what and when* of cancer. Rather, when cancer does occur, we must make the best of it.

As paradigms of human cancer, let us construct a model of the disease, interspersed with pertinent biologic data, in (a) any one of the three cancer surgeons, Mayo, Wilkie and Borges (Chapter 1), who died of cancer of the stomach; (b) Aldous Huxley, who fell victim to a cancer of the tongue; [37] (c) Lenore Schwartz, a young Chicago scholar, artist and teacher who died of leukemia at the age of 23, and in whose name the Lenore Schwartz Leukemia Research Foundation at Florida was established, [38] and (d) John Gunther, Jr., who died of a brain cancer while still in his teens. [39]

The inception of the cancer, in each person listed above, was as a very small, silent event that predeterminedly affected, at one or more places, a small number of cells – cells that were originally normal. The newly formed cancerous cells started multiplying, but no faster than normal cells as was hitherto thought. This slowness of cancer cells' proliferation, in comparison with the rate of proliferation of normal cells, confirmed over a wide range of cancers, [6, 40, 98, 258, 315] has led to the suggestion [40] that cancer be better regarded as a disease of cell-accumulation rather than of rapid proliferation.

A cancer cell measures no larger than a normal cell – one-hundredth of a millimeter across. This sheer micro-size of a cancer cell accounts for the fact that, following the inception of cancer, it must have ordinarily taken several years before the cancer bothered these individuals, or came to the attention of their doctors. On the basis of the modern cytokinetic studies, it has been computed that any cancer, before causing symptoms or striking the eyes of the clinician, takes anything from two to seventeen years – $2\frac{1}{2}$ years for a rapidly fatal cancer as of the lung to seventeen years for breast cancer. And during this interval, there is no instrumental, immunological, or biochemical method that

25

could detect this microscopic focus of growing cancer, be it the amazingly sophisticated tomography,[308] or the quantitative imaging[311] designed to synchronously scan up to 250 parallel transverse cross-sections of the human body. A cancer just one cubic mm in size is worth at least 1,000,000 cells.[41] Any diagnosable cancer is thus, at least a-million-cell-worth, and many years old, with twenty-four hours of each day of each year at its disposal to leave the starting point and go and lodge elsewhere in the blissfully unaware individual.[42]

Let us be happy that the six luminaries of our story were not deprived of the much-sought-and-advertised 'early-diagnosis' for want of the latest computer off the IBM assembly line. As far back as in 1927, Cheatle,[43] writing in the *British Medical Journal* declared that 'when a lump appears in the carcinoma, the disease is well advanced, and is already threatening the patient's life, possibly beyond all hopes of cure.' What Cheatle said of breast cancer in 1927, Logan[12] repeated in 1975, with the question – is there anything like an early cancer?

In Mayo, Wilkie and Huxley, the discovery of the tumour was sudden, and until that time they neither had the knowledge of it, nor any problems. They were operated, unrewardingly. Borges, a humanitarian as we knew him, was feeling uneasy for some time, but he took it as gastric upset and continued to work; then, one day, he was investigated and operated upon. Borges lived and worked for many months after that until the spread caused obstructive jaundice to which he succumbed, with dignity. A few months before his death, he delivered an oration at Pune (Maharashtra State), India, and a part of the oration is reproduced here, courtesy of Lt. Dr. Bhagwat, lately of the Armed Forces Medical College, Pune: 'I have treated thousands of cases surgically, radiologically and by cytotoxic drugs. A number of times people met me later and

26

said, "Doctor, if I knew I was going to live like this, I would not have come to you." I have rarely failed to diagnose a case when the disease was not quite controllable! I have left the disease and removed the patient in many cases. I have succeeded in leaving behind a trail of family-malnutrition and many of their children without education. I have now come to the conclusion that, let us in every case ask whether it is not wiser to leave the patient to be released by death than to try to relieve him by surgery; cure is only a dream yet!'

What Borges emphasized, on the eve of his long career as a cancerologist, was the *cacotelic* nature of cancer therapy. (*cacotelic*, from Greek, means *tending to end badly*). Gius[259, 260] introduced this term to drive home an important cancerologic lesson: 'Operations intended to palliate (or even cure) may sometimes make the patient worse than he was initially.' The modern cancerologists ought to take a cue from the foregoing, and be publicly candid about cancer therapy. But they won't. As one senior scientist of the *National Cancer Institute* confessed: 'It just doesn't pay to rock the boat.'[44]

The course of Ms. Schwartz's illness is not available to the authors, but a fair guess can be made. The possibility that for quite some time she must have been blissfully free of *any* symptoms may be realized from the recently established fact that in leukemia, when there is complete remission, a patient's bone marrow has at least a 1000 million cells.[45, 265] At some stage then her leukemia could have turned from the silent to the clinical stage. She could have had fever or a sore throat, or felt weak or out-of-sorts; then came the blood counts and the frightening diagnosis of leukemia was established.

What treatment must she have received? X-ray therapy and/or chemotherapy, both greater enemies to many a normal cell from head-to-foot, bowel to bone marrow.

Lenore's leukemic count must have gone down, to the academic satisfaction of her doctors, but so must have her vitality, resistance and hemoglobin. Eventually, Lenore succumbed, we do not know to what – the disease or the treatment! Many a leukemia gets controlled, but the patient dies. Perhaps, it may be argued, had she lived, or had had her leukemia now, her bone marrow, the seat of the leukemic process, could have been first destroyed completely by very heavy doses of toxic drugs and X-rays, rendering it thus free of *any* cells, cancerous or normal. The now-completely-defenceless patient could have been grafted with bone marrow from another human to give the patient white/red blood cells indispensable for survival, as also hopefully to give donor-lymphocytes that would act against any residual leukemia. But such superheroic measures have proved tragically futile: twenty-four leukemic cases were grafted.[46] In seven cases, the graft failed to survive, and the patients died with 'aplasia' or completely cell-less bone marrow. In seventeen, the graft succeeded only to unleash a vicious attack on the host – ' "the graft-versus-host disease (GVHD)" which is particularly severe in man'[46] – to kill thirteen patients, ten in no time, two after some time, and one a little later. The remaining four with successful graft died with 'controlled' GVHD and recurrent leukemia. The foregoing problems reported[46] in 1969 remain essentially unchanged today, in 1978.[272-275]

The saga[39] of John Gunther Jr. is too well-known to be described here. The brave boy was treated with the most advanced allopathic and the most hopeful naturopathic measures, but to no avail. The fault wasn't with the treatment but with the cancer. All brain cancers, even when they appear 'benign' to the microscopists have, what Willis[20] calls, a 'wide field of origin.' You remove it at one place, and the next one grows for recognition, and may be removed. In the end, the cancer wins, for want of sacrifice-able brain.

The true-to-life stories above may appear grim and selective. One could as well have picked up eminent people who did very well – pathologist-author Boyd, Alexander Solzhenitsyn, Sigmud Freud, John Wayne. But the essential sequence of events remains the same, whether the cancer is benign or otherwise. The most important moral, if there may be any, of the above accounts is that cancer is mercifully quiet and unobtrusive for many years after its inception. And there lies the benignancy of this malignant process.

There are some more human issues confounded by the seeming vagaries of cancer. 'Why me, when I never smoked, and why not my friend who always did?' Cancer affects more-or-less a fixed percentage of the herd, and it all depends where one gets caught in this probability distri-bution. Of those who get it, the age at which cancer occurs is *normally* distributed so that the one gets it at 19, the other at 39 and the third at 93. Such distribution holds true both for overall cancer and for cancer at one particular site.

Some cancers allow a longer lease of life, with no treatment or minimal treatment while others, of the same histological variety, prove rapidly fatal despite timely and adequate treatment. The secret of this lies in the cancer itself, the survival-time itself being *normally* distributed, thus accounting for the early death of Karnofsky the cancer-specialist, and a long active life for John Wayne, the Hollywood hero, both having had cancer of the lung. Such unpredictable autonomy of cancers has led cancerologists to classify, albeit *a posteriori*, cancers as *good*, and *bad*, the former amenable to *any* treatment, the latter to none.[3] In a larger perspective, the *goodness* or *badness* resides not so much even in cancer itself, as much as in the helplessly unpredictable nature of any individual's biological trajectory.

What Makes Cancer Incurable?

The real enemy of cancer cure is not the cancer itself, but the adjacent normal cell, waiting for its turn to grow cancerous.

In cancerologic parlance, this process of a normal cell joining the cancerous troop is called *recruitment*. The cancerous army thus can potentially become as big as that of the normal cells in the body. This simple fact rules out the cancerologist's dream of 'The Last Surviving Cancer Cell: The Chances of Killing It.'[47] That is not all. While surgery's fault lies in spreading[246, 247] a cancer which was localized, X-ray therapy[6, 248, 249] and chemotherapy[6, 8, 15, 101, 102, 250] are agencies recognized for their ability to induce normal cells to cancerate faster: 'The carcinogenic activity of many of our chemotherapeutic agents is now under advisement.'[250] Chemotherapy can render[251] berserk a benignantly behaving malignancy, and be effective to the point of being lethal: 'The aggressive chemotherapeutic approach used . . . is often lethal to the patient with LRE (Leukemic Reticulo-Endotheliosis, a type of leukemia).'[252]

The only human cancer that does not present this Damoclean demeanor of recruitment is the rare gestational choriocarcinoma that occurs in women following pregnancy. But this is so, because it is a cancer 'transferred'[20] from the fetus to the mother, thus not being autochthonous, or springing from the mother's own tissues. Naturally such a cancer allows a complete cure, for after 'the last cancer cell,' there are no normal cells to recruit. This is, as yet, the solitary triumph of cancer chemotherapy, for reasons that reside exclusively in the cancer.

FOUR

CAUSELESS AND UNPREVENTABLE

THE medical finger accuses almost everything as cancer-ogenic *and having accused, moves on to accuse* still more. From the time Percival Pott suggested the relationship between soot and scrotal cancer in chimney-sweeps, the central theme in cancerology has been the postulated causal relationship between cancerogens and cancerogenesis, an endless search for the culprit cancerogens[48, 49] resulting in a publication explosion that fills innumerable pages in scientific cancer literature. Very few thinkers have raised any objection against the search for cancerogens which is really like asking a blind man to go into a dark room to find a black hat which is not there. A certain note of disdain may be seen in Kaplan's[50] words: 'I would like to question just why it is desirable to find more cancerogens when we already seem to be plagued with them?' The cancerogens that we know about, from experimental and clinical data, are by now legion. Boyd[51] poses a simple question, as to how, with cancerogens all around us, most of us escape?

The latest accused is the human sperm, with the charge that, apart from occasionally fertilizing human ova, it fertilizes the cells of the cervix in the female to induce the much-feared cancer of the cervix.[52] Thus arises the sweeping conclusion that 'untold numbers of husbands bear some measure of responsibility for initiating malignancies (cancers) in untold numbers of wives.'[22] Should a woman with cancer of the cervix sue her present/former husband/lover for having given the wrong sperm? Hypothetical as this may seem, it may become a reality today.[53]

The gains of this rabid cancerogenism have been nil; the harm done is a global cancerophobia; should people eat, drink, breathe, or make love. 'Unfortunately, when it comes to cancer, American society (and the many societies which follow, as a matter of faith) is far from rational.'[10] For this state of panic, fear, irrationality, and paranoia -- 'CANCER! ALARM! CANCER!' – gripping us all, Ingelfinger[10] blames doctors, cancer societies, and of course, the media who specialize in converting all the trivia on cancer into sensational matters.

How do we cure ourselves of this? The voluminous and evergrowing statistics on cancerogens cannot be matched by counter-statistics. Inundated by the floodtide of cancerogens, no one has been bold enough to perceive and proclaim the very absurdity of anything and everything maliciously cancerizing mankind. The burden of the disproof is on the disbeliever. If a claim is made that drinking tea or running at the Olympics causes cancer, the possibilities are only two – right, or wrong. The 'rightness' of the proposition depends on the claimer's conviction and some statistical data. The 'wrongness' has to be proved beyond doubt, without taking recourse to statistics. For, till such time that some statistics favourable to the proposition exist, the counter-statistics are connived at by scientists and people biased in favour of the *causation* of cancer.

However, where statistics cannot help, logic can. The proposition that a cancerogen causes a cancer is invalidated by the latter occurring without, and refusing to occur despite, the former. This *conundrum of a cancer-causalist* could be expressed as follows: X causes Y, but why does Y occur without, and not occur despite, X?

No cancerogen has yet proved to be *causa sine qua non* of any particular cancer, in humans or in animals, *in vivo* or *in vitro*. Citing Hume, Fuller[54] puts down, as the earmark of causality, an *invariant relation* of events in which the cause must *precede* its effect and the effect must follow its cause, in time. 'It is this sense of *must* which distinguishes causal connection from coincidence'.[54] Further, Fuller[54] emphasizes, the effect must immediately follow the cause: 'Causality can no more jump gaps in time than it can gaps in space.' The concept of 'latency'[55] that allows as many as thirty-six years between the exposure to the postulated cause and the occurrence of cancer is, because of the irreconcilable temporal gap, clearly against the causalism of cancerogenism.

This brings us to the Bombay razor (cf. the one proposed by William of Occam): *Any causalistic proposition that A causes B must in the same breath explain how A fails to cause B, and how B manages to occur without A.* To take but one example, the authenticated statistics are that on an average, of 740 smokers, one gets lung cancer.[56] Such being the case, the onus of proving/explaining how cancer failed to occur is, for the causalists, 739 times greater than to prove how it did. No causalistic proposition, be it heart disease, hypertension, or cancer, has been able to meet the logical sharpness of the Bombay razor. No wonder the causes keep on changing, like ladies' fashions. For cancer of the cervix, for example, it was smegma yesterday, but is sperm today. For lung cancer, too, smoking is going out, and some unexplained predisposition is coming in. And this parade will continue till we accept the universal *intrinsicality* of cancer.

Way back in 1918, Bertrand Russell[57] delivered a devastating judgement against causalism: 'All philosophers, of every school, imagine that causation is one of the fundamental axioms of science, yet oddly enough, in advanced sciences such as gravitational astronomy, the word cause never occurs.' Causalism survives, nay thrives in medicine probably because either it is not science, or it is not advanced or it isn't both. Russell[57] gives some other reason for its survival: 'The law of causality, I believe, like much that passes muster among philosophers, is a relic of a bygone age, surviving, like the monarchy, only because it is erroneously supposed to do no harm.' Cancerological causalism, having presented mankind with hysterical cancerophobia, marches on regardless. This is despite the fact that even the much-vaunted virus and smoking have lost their cancerogenic value. Viruses have been held as lab artifacts that have nothing to do with human cancer[5], and smoking has aptly been declared as the leading cause of statistics.[58]

Koestler[59] has alluded to the perversity of scientists. Such perversity reaches its climax when patients are purportedly 'cured' by the very agents known as causing cancer – irradiation, chemicals, and hormones. Viruses and immunity had hitherto escaped this cancerological diabolism of *what causes, cures* cancer. However, viruses have been mooted as curative[60] while immunity, our last hope against cancer, has been incriminated[61] as not only cancerogenic, but also cancerotrophic. Diagnostic procedures (mammography[62] right now) are not exempt from the cancerogenic scare. All that is done to cure cancer, appears to cause cancer.

The noble aim behind the hunt for the cause is the promise of the prevention. 'Since so little is known about the origin and development of neoplasia, it is not surprising that many cancers can be neither prevented nor cured.'[63] What if much is known? Reviewing a book ambitiously titled *The*

34

Prevention of Cancer, Jelliffe[64] concluded that, although the various authors provide an excellent analysis of the large amount of data related to the *causation* of different cancers, no reasonable means are provided anywhere for prevention. 'For example,' Jellife[64] remarked, 'after twelve erudite pages on breast cancer, the reader can discover no practical alternative to prophylactic bilateral mastectomy at an early age.' Harvey Cushing[65] exclaimed that, like many other catchwords, *prevention* can be overworked: 'There is only one ultimate and effectual preventive for the maladies to which flesh is heir, and that is death.' Life's close link with cancer means that the only way to prevent cancer is to prevent life. And, in a way, the only truly effective remedy for cancer is death.

The realization that cancer is not *caused*, and therefore, is not *'preventable'* is a mixed blessing. The happy part is that the all-pervasive cancerophobia will disappear and we shall be able to sip coffee and enjoy a smoke without the subconscious feeling of committing slow suicide, by inviting cancer. The bitter part is that some of us – one in five – would always be doomed to cancer, no matter what. Sad? But that is how Nature operates.

FIVE

NOT DIAGNOSABLE, NOR EARLY ENOUGH

T HE aim of cancer diagnosis is to circumscribe the cancer completely, or as the therapists desire, to go well beyond it to ensure the efficacy of treatment, and thus provide a cure. This seemingly simple task has maintained its Sisyphean character for the following, essentially biological, reasons:

1. Cancer is a disease of the whole organism:[17] Having started at one place, cancer imperceptibly involves the whole body of an individual by also spreading to, and colonizing, many more areas in the body. Whenever the cancer acquires a sufficient bulk at the original (primary) site and/or at the subsequent (secondary/metaststic) sites, it forms and presents itself as a lump, or a tumour.

2. By the time a cancer presents itself to the clinician, it is many-cells-strong, and usually many-sites-strong.

3. What the clinician looks for, or can look for, is the formation of a lump, popularly called a tumour (L. *tumere*, to swell).

4. The acceptance of the tumour as *the diagnosis* is *ipso facto* the admission of diagnostic defeat. It is tantamount to noticing only the proverbial tip of the iceberg.

5. There is no escape from the conclusion that 'the clinician, even if he diagnoses cancer at the earliest possible stage, is dealing only with the late stages of a disease process.'[17] The *lateness* is not just a matter of time, but of space, the cancer having gone well beyond the circumscribing capacity of the diagnostician. No wonder, time is not of the essence in cancer diagnosis, 'late' cases often outliving the 'early' ones. 'The survival-rates after different periods of delay before seeking medical advice often show a curious paradox' – 'the greater the delay and the longer the history of symptoms, the greater was the survival-rate.'[66]

6. The proof of all our diagnosing lies in our gaining ground against cancer. The facts point otherwise. What we therefore achieve is a pseudodiagnosis which has refused to change its character no matter what gadgetry is at our disposal.

Attempts at detecting a cancer even before the appearance of any symptoms[261, 262] have proved futile: 'In a group of sixteen cases in which esophageal cancer was diagnosed prior to the development of symptoms while the patient was under active medical surveillance, Palmer could demonstrate no improvement in survival.'[261] An editorial[42] in *The New England Journal of Medicine* crisply commented: ' "Early" is an adjective of *time* – not of size, dissemination or clinical manifestations. Yet, enslaved by medical semantics, too many people equate "early" with small, localized, asymptomatic (or minimally productive of symptoms'.

37

What about those cancers that are truly early in the temporal sense? Here, too, the situation is unredeeming: *The Lancet* editorialized[66] that 'the stage of disease is a function not of time, but of the (inherent) tumour type.'

7. Clinical cancerology runs on the illusion that tumour-diagnosis is equivalent to cancer-diagnosis. This is an act of great faith, both of the clinician and of the patient. This faith accounts for, what Wilfred Trotter called, *the mysterious viability of the false*.

8. What the diagnostician really achieves, is to locate the area where the cancer *dis-eases* the individual, while the submerged part of the cancerous iceberg remains unseen. A clinician's ability to locate the site and nature of this *dis-ease*, and the ability to ease the condition, is the brightest and the most indispensable part of clinical practice.

9. Cancerophobia and indifference to the biology of cancer conspire to induce a clinician to err towards the false-positive diagnosis.

10. Efforts have been made to catch a cancer before it dares to be a cancer, by detecting 'precancer.' The whole science of precancer is marred by ambivalence – semantic and microscopic.

Both 9 and 10 lead to, what Park and Lees[67] called, *pragmatic diagnosis*, detailed below:

(i) 'Pragmatically diagnosed cancer' is 'probably not cancer, but safer away' type of approach.[67] This consists of diagnosing a lump as cancer, merely to play safe.

(ii) In 1923, Bloodgood,[68] from his experiences at Johns Hopkins over thirty-three years in retrospect, wrote of 'Benign Lumps Diagnosed Cancer or Suspicious of Cancer.' Bloodgood[68] remarked that during the thirty-three years of observations, the above group had been seen with increas-

ing frequency in the laboratory – with breasts that were the seat of chronic cystic mastitis, tuberculosis, encapsulated adenomas, or cysts with an intracystic papilloma having been diagnosed as carcinoma. Such a group of cases – relatively quite large – when classed with unequivocal carcinomas, increased the percentage of five-year cures and made it impossible to correctly assess the controllable factor (of preoperative duration) in the cure of cancer. Bloodgood[68] concluded the topic with an objective and far-reaching generalization: 'As this element of error has been present in my own investigations for years, I feel justified in the conclusion that it is present in all statistical studies throughout the world.'

(iii) In 1951, Park and Lees[67] diagnosed the pragmatism prevalent in cancerology whereby non-cancers were declared as cancers to inflate the cure-rates.

(iv) In 1954, McKinnon[69] stated: 'Today it is a safe generalization that all competent cytologists and pathologists agree that, in histopathology, there is no sharp line dividing malignancy and non-malignancy. But, in practice, the division is made sharply, as it must be, in all cases presenting, and naturally and unavoidably, with the diagnoses tending to the positive rather than the negative side.'

(v) In 1968, Cowdry[263] detected, from extensive epidemiologic studies, the mysterious 'paradox of increasing incidence and decreasing mortality rates' of carcinoma cervix. By 1974, *carcinoma in situ* of cervix was reported as 100% cured.[264]

(vi) In 1973, such pragmatism meant 690,000 hysterectomies performed in a year in the USA, many 'unnecessarily!'[70]

(vii) With nothing else changed, such pragmatism meant a sudden, nearly four-fold, leap in cancer rates for the year 1975.[48]

39

(viii) In 1977, a coordinated study of breast cancer, between the NCI and the ACS in the USA, revealed[204] that as many as sixty-six women were diagnosed to have cancer when there was none, and another twenty-two were branded as having cancer, when in reality the microscopic basis was 'unclear'; all these women were operated upon because of the cancer-diagnosis.

In a militantly litigant society, the pathologist and the clinician are wont to play safe. The credit is theirs if a non-cancer removed as cancer, yields a 'cure'. Moreover, the 'safe away' approach also promotes surgery, as evinced from *(vi)* above.

Microscope Unreliable in Cancer/Precancer Diagnosis

From all the cancerologic experience the world has had, one could generalize that *a cancer cell may be defined as one that has proved itself by behaving as such*. There is no cellular feature that can help predict that such and such a cell will, at or after such and such a time, behave as cancerous – namely, proliferate unrestrainedly to form a mass/tumour and/or spread from its site of origin to other organs. Cancer cytologists and histologists (experts who pass the judgement of cancer on the basis of microscopic features of cells and tissues) rely on the usually taken for granted features such as cell size, nuclear size/shape, cellular arrangement, and so on, but such judgements betray their falsity and unreliability when 'cancerous' tissues behave noncancerously and *vice versa*. Notwithstanding this appalling state of ambivalence in the field of cancer, cancerologists have chosen to use the proved-unreliable cellular criteria to spawn the new science of precancer.

Cancerologists and cancer societies, so vociferous on the issues they champion, have almost deliberately failed to educate the public on how unreliable the judgement of cancer/precancer passed on a lesion under the microscope can be. Cytological research has revealed the cancer cell to be no distinctive structural entity, but an organ of behaviour (see para above). Smithers[71] in an attack on cytologism, generalized that 'there is no such thing as a cancer cell – only cells behaving in a manner arbitrarily defined as being cancerous.' This observation has been amply vindicated by many a cancer refusing to declare itself as cancer under the microscope.[20, 72] Despite this unreliability of the microscopic view, the almost universal concepts of benignancy and malignancy are based on the microscopic features, as typified by the statement that 'many cerebral tumours, histologically benign, are biologically malignant.'[73] Similarly, many lesions, histologically malignant, are biologically benign.[20, 74] Histologically provable prostatic cancer is present in a high percentage (30%) of men above 50 years of age. A majority of these cancers (28.6%) act *benign* – they do not kill.[75] 'The startling discrepancy,' *The Lancet* editorialized, 'between the clinical and post-mortem prevalence of prostatic carcinoma has virtually demolished ideas of cancer as an essentially killing disease.'[74]

Precancer

While cancer itself went begging for microscopic definition, cancerologists opened up an altogether new field called precancer, a sort of earlier-than-early cancer. Applied extensively to the cervix of the uterus and the breasts, in females, the science relies on examining cells and tissues and grading them regarding their assumed proximity to cancer, or otherwise. The terms frequently used are dysplasia, carcinoma-in-situ (meaning cancer-in-its-place, without any spread elsewhere), precancer, and minimal cancer.

The diagnostic measures used for the cervix are cytology,

41

histopathology, and colposcopy. Cervical cytology was initiated by George Papanicolaou and the technique is mostly referred to as Pap smear – a thriving industry by itself. For the breast, histopathology is assisted by mammography, xerography and thermography, all of which aim at locating 'suspicious' areas in the breast.

The semantic ambivalence, reflecting the conceptual confusion is enormous: 'This terminological difficulty is greater in gynaecological pathology than in any other chapter on pathology, different authors using one and the same term in a different sense.'[76] The unreliability of Pap smear may be gauged from the incidence of reported 'malignancy' ranging from 33% to 100% and 5% to 60% in the same grades of smears.[52] The histopathologic descriptions of carcinoma-in-situ of the cervix are as many as the publications on it.[77] Siegler[78] sent the histopathologic slides of cervical precancer to twenty-five different pathologists and their interpretations betrayed 'disconcerting' variations and disagreements in the fundamental evaluations. Colposcopy, for detecting cervical precancer, has been characterized by Way[79] as 'the biggest gynaecological hoax of this or any other century.' Needless to say, the ambivalent situation – semantic and microscopic – is no different *vis-à-vis* the assumed *precancer* above the female umbilicus, i.e., of the breasts.

And what does all this microscopic uncertainty in the field of cancer lead to? 'Uncertainty is resolved by doing more: the patient asks for more, the doctor orders more.'[80] And this in cancerology means far more diagnoses than are warranted. It has not as yet been appreciated, that as much as cancer can be left untreated, it can be left undiagnosed as well. And there lies a cure for the paralyzing cancerophobia. Fischer[81] has a point here: 'Do you ever ponder the advisability of *not* making a diagnosis and thereby avoiding a death sentence?'

SIX

NOT CURABLE, HIGHLY PALLIATABLE

T HE *raison d'être* of cancer therapy is that the chief clinical
manifestation of cancer is a mass of cells – a celluloma
called a tumour or a lump. A cancer therapist's knowledge
begins with a tumour, and ends with it. By a variety of
measures, the tumour or the lump can be made to disappear. The whole cycle of detection and destruction of the
lump is repeated on the reappearance of the lump. It is a
sobering thought that cancer therapy is nothing more than
glorified 'lumpology'.

Tumour and Before

As elaborated earlier, both the patient and the doctor are
blissfully unaware of all the happenings, till such time as the
tumour dis-eases the owner or is detected by the doctor. It is
all *ignorance* from the start of cancer up to the time of
detection of the tumour.

43

Tumour and After

What, once the tumour is found and removed? Back to *ignorance* again for some inescapable reasons: The incurable individuality of each cancer and of its owner make unpredictable, (a) what the cancer will now do to the patient, and (b) what the treatment will do to the cancer. Regarding the former, the course may be, like for the celebrities listed in Chapter 3, inexorably downhill, despite all possible measures. Or, as for the pathologist-author Boyd[51], the tumour may not reappear for a lifetime.

Treatment, in fact, may aggravate the cancer: Even after considering the most painstaking criteria of operability, there are women in whom surgery manages to accelerate the evolution of breast cancer[82]. Surgical intervention may markedly precipitate distant spread, so that 'surgical intervention must be excluded as the first therapeutic step, even in stage I breast cancer.'[83] Surgery, the oldest, most widely employed, and relatively the most innocuous of all measures, is itself beset with such unpredictable hazards. What then could one say of radiotherapy and chemotherapy with their indiscriminate cytotoxic and 'marrow-devastating'[84] potential?

Treated, *the tumour is out, the cancer is not,* much less the cancerability of normal tissues. Over a century ago, Billroth[85] aphorized that surgery removes a tumour, but not the patient's diathesis for cancer. 'Unfortunately it must be admitted that all cancer surgery is in large measure palliative, given the occult spread of the disease before treatment in a high percentage of cases.'[86] The much-celebrated victory over leukemia must contend with the fact that, although by definition the peripheral blood picture and the bone marrow are *normal* during complete remission, 100 million to 1000 million leukemic cells still remain, making relapse inevitable[45].

44

Whither Cancer Treatment?

Thus, all told, prior to the detection of and after the detection/treatment of a tumour, clinicians are still almost know-nothings.

Glemser's worldwide survey of *Man Against Cancer*[22] only revealed that the realistic title of his book could have been *Man Helpless Against Cancer:* Surgery was declared dispensable, radiotherapy obsolete, and chemotherapy a farce. In 1969 talk of treating cancer was tantamount to Ecclesiastes' *Vanitas vanitatum*: 'Nothing is worth doing, no way is better than another.'[87] Has real progress been made?

'At the present time,' Brooke[88] generalized in 1971, 'cancer treatment appears to have reached a culmination, a peak beyond which we have not moved for several decades.' But as all of the therapeutic measures against cancer, as of today, are held dispensable, we are forced to conclude that what cancer therapy reached was its Peterian[150] (cf. Peter principle zenith of imperfection 'several decades' ago, and all that we have been doing is to move in circles and call it 'progress,' 'recent advances' and so on. Such euphemisms may be justified on the geometric ground that all circular motions are made up of a series of motions in a straight line, and any straight line motion implies progress.

Cancer therapy has almost entirely betrayed the application of lumpolytic logic to the false premise of a cure. Watts[89] has described the peculiar and perhaps fatal fallacy of modern times: *the confusion of symbol with reality*. Such fallacy dominates cancerology so that what is diagnosed and treated is not cancer – 'a disease of the whole organism'[17] – but merely its most evident manifestation, a lump, or an *-oma*. The consoling cures obtained are 'largely limited to some unusual forms of malignant disease, such as chorionic epithelioma (gestational choriocarcinoma) in women'[90], being a function of the nature of the cancer, rather than due to any ingenuity of the hit-and-

45

miss treatment.

And Yet Cancer Must Be Treated

However, the indispensable role of cancer therapy must be emphasized. Despite the accepted impotence of all therapies against autochthonous cancer, one and all measures are useful when employed to ease a dis-eased cancer patient. A cancer patient with a blocked gullet or intestinal obstruction, a mass in the brain, a massive ungainly jaw from Burkitt's tumour, a fungating mass in the breast, or a large sarcoma of the bone cannot be subjected to a course on the philosophy of whither cancer therapy, but must be eased immediately with an appropriate palliative measure. Cancer will be with mankind forever, being a part, and progenitor of it. Cancer therapists will be needed to play their vital palliative role as long as mankind survives.

With this background, we can now draw some generalizations on cancer therapy.

1. Cancer, a process characterized by accumulation of newly formed cells, dis-eases an individual when it forms a mass or a tumour large enough to obtrude on the physiology or the psyche of the patient. Equally, it comes to the stage of diagnosability by the doctor, *only* when it is many million cells strong and quite a few years old. The therapy of cancer, except for the 'gestational choriocarcinoma,' is always a *palliative* measure.

2. A cancer's manifestation may be (a) restricted locally as a lump in the tongue, esophagus, brain or on the arm, (b) also found regionally as when a tongue cancer spreads to the lymph nodes in the neck, or (c) all over the body – 'systemic disease' – as in blood cancers, lumph node

46

cancers and some cancers such as melanoma that have spread all over.

3. Cancer present as a local and/or regional mass is most amenable to being cut away by surgery, usually together with a fair margin of healthy tissues. Most cancers so present themselves and are so treated. Surgery – conservative, radical or supraradical – is the sheet-anchor of cancer therapy. 'The surgical removal of malignant tumours is the oldest form of treatment for this condition, has retained its leading role in the course of centuries and is still the treatment of choice in a high percentage of cases.'[91]

4. Systemic or whole-body cancers, such as blood cancers (leukemias), Hodgkin's disease, other lymphomas, may be managed by systemic or whole-body measures such as X-ray therapy and cell-poisons euphemistically called anti-cancer drugs. Cancers starting locally – melanoma, lining of the uterus, intestine – may spread to various sites in the body so that the treatment has to be given as for systemic cancers.

5. Some cancers, as of the breast, thyroid, prostate, re-spond, *albeit* unpredictably and temporarily[15], to admini-stration of hormones and/or ablation of glands secreting hormones.

6. In all leading centres, a combination of therapeutic measures is usually employed. The advantage of surgery is a total absence of toxic action on other cells; its limitation is its limited reach. X-ray therapy and chemotherapy provide an all-body reach; their outstanding limitation is the toll they take of the many cell-populations that divide faster than many a cancer. The common result is – the hair falls off, the mouth, intestine and skin ulcerate, and the patient becomes pale and defenseless because of depression of the bone marrow.

47

7. The follow-up insisted upon by cancer therapists is to watch for *recurrence* of the lump (or the heightened cell count as in leukemias). The logical sequence to recurrence is treatment, all over again. Sigmund Freud had thirty-three operations for his oral cancer, over a period of sixteen years[36].

8. The science of cancer therapy does not exclude such measures as analgesics, stronger pain-killers as morphine, transfusions, dietary supplements and so on so as to make the patient feel better.

9. It may be difficult to realize that one of the most fruitful measures in cancer therapy is an attack on the *I-worry tower* of the patient – the tower crumbles against the power of a positive approach. 'The victims of this disease,' Weil[92] aphorized as far back as 1915, 'seem to be in a very high degree "suggestible" and impressionable and respond nobly to every therapeutic effort.' Issels' experience seems to bear out Weil's observation: 'In the twenty years of experience with the so-called incurables, I have seen what reservoirs of undreamt-of strength and courage can be drawn upon, even in "terminal" cases by the adoption of a positive attitude.'[93] Lewin[94] has talked of a physician needing the ability to manage his own anxiety against cancer; what *kills* a patient often is the everything-is-lost attitude of his physician which is betrayed in his eyes, words, tone or even in the way he walks towards the patient's bed.

Cure-rates in Cancer Therapy

With average survival not extending beyond three to five years for the majority of cancers treated by the best hands in the best centres, it has become imperative to talk of five year, ten year, and twenty year *cure rates, albeit* at the level of a group of patients *similarly treated for a supposedly similar disease*. In an age when it is advocated that the patient should be fully apprised of the gravity of his disease, the severity of the treatment, and the unpredictability of the outcome, it is as well that the patient is told that his survival is a *herd function* ranging from three months to thirty years, and that his own survival would depend on what place he occupies, through probability distribution, on the herd survival curve.

'When it comes to appraising the effectiveness of treatment,' Sutherland[95] comments, 'one of the difficulties is the striking range in the natural duration of cancer of the same site in a series of cases.' Sutherland[95] gives among many cancers, the natural duration of cancers (left untreated) of the tongue and oral cavity in males ranging from three months to seventy-five months, and of the *cervix uteri* and female breast, from three months to twelve and a half years and two months to seventeen and a half years respectively.

The most commonly cited five year survival rate as a standard of cure is comparative and fallacious assuming as it must that all the cases 'if untreated would have a nil per cent five year survival rate.'[67] *The real cure rate*, Park and Lees[67] define, is represented by the difference between the five year survival rate of all cases following treatment and the five year survival rate of those same cases had they been left untreated. 'In several forms of cancer, survival for five years after a therapeutic procedure means little by itself, since a considerable proportion of untreated patients are known to survive five years or longer.'[96] Park and Lees[67], in a detailed, highly critical article entitled, 'The absolute curability of cancer of the breast,' and containing numerous graphs and mathematical calculations, concluded that (a) it could not be proved that the survival rate of breast cancer, using as an index the five year survival rate, was in any way affected by treatment, (b) treatment was quite

49

ineffective in reducing the mortality from metastatic spread, and (c) if the treatment was 'in any way' effective, the so-called effectiveness could not exceed that required to increase the overall five year survival rate by more than 5% to 10%.

The whole business of five year, ten year and x-year survival rates is marred by the fallacy of an early or late 'countdown.'[97] Ms. A has a breast lump, and she does not bother about it for four years. Then she decides to get it treated, and dies after two years, to be registered as a case that came late and, therefore, died early. Ms. B has a similar lump, she gets treated within six months, lives for four years, and is registered, in contrast to Ms. A, as the case that came earlier and survived longer. In reality, Ms. A lived with her cancer for six years, and Ms. B for four and a half years. The apparent longer survival of Ms. B was because the countdown on her started earlier. An extended limitation of the above fallacy of countdown arises from the fact that no one – neither the patient nor the doctor – knows exactly when the cancer started in the body.

A cancer patient, at an individual level, is no statistic, as he is often made out to be. Carrying within himself two forms of uniqueness, one his own and the other that of the cancer he carries, he does not lend himself to any fruitful predictions or comparisons.

Victory Over Childhood Leukemia

The current showpiece[14, 22, 271] of the cancer world is the hard-won victory over an otherwise rapidly fatal leukemia of children, called the acute lymphoblastic leukemia, usually abbreviated as ALL. Firstly, we may see the nature of the success and then understand its mechanism.

(i) Before the introduction of 'effective' therapy, the average survival rate was less than three months; now a small percentage of patients survive five years and more. The continuing survival of an ALL patient, under therapy, with disappearance of leukemic cells from the bone marrow and blood, is generally called 'remission,' a term applicable to other forms of leukemia as well.

(ii) Leukemic cells persist during remission, for the disease rapidly recurs on discontinuation of therapy: 'It has been estimated that before treatment the cancer patient has about 10^{12} (1000 billion) or more malignant cells in his body, and that when he is brought into so-called complete remission he still has from 10^9 (one billion) to 10^{10} (10 billion) viable malignant cells.' [265]

(iii) The observed increases in average survival, therefore, reflect only improved palliation.

(iv) The most important factor in survival is not the type of leukemic cells nor their pretreatment number, but the response to therapy – a factor that unpredictably resides in an individual patient and his cancer, and *not* in the treatment. Under the same therapy, boys may fare significantly[269] worse than girls.

(v) The treatment accorded to ALL cases is no different from that given in other forms of leukemia, or cancers. The treatment comprises agents – drugs, X-rays – that act as cancer-inducing agents in the laboratory, and sometimes in humans. The complications of the therapy of ALL are as varied and formidable as with other cancers. Despite remission, patients die – seemingly not of leukemia, but of infections of the most unusual nature by micro-organisms that are ordinarily non-pathogenic, or of sudden hemorrhage.

(vi) Therapy of ALL produces remission possibly by

pushing the disease, as it were, under the carpet. While the therapy is busy providing remission by clearing the bone marrow and blood of leukemic cells, leukemic cells settle in the brain, spinal cord, meninges, testes etc., to eventually bring about the so-called extramedullary (outside the bone marrow) relapse. Certain drugs[268] probably assist such transfer of the disease from the bone marrow to elsewhere.

(vii) ALL therapy is essentially a titration between killing more leukemic cells while hoping to kill less of normal cells.[315] No known treatment of ALL has such selective action.[98] Drugs and X-rays exercise relentless toxicity, and the leukemic cells commonly turn resistant to the action of drugs.

(viii) Newer methods[271–275, 315] of treating ALL are afoot – varied types of immunotherapy, and bone marrow trans-plantation. The formidable problems posed by transplan-tation – 'a harrowing method of treatment'[275] – are nowhere near a solution, and present a highly nocuous double-edge: The transplantee must be pre-prepared to accept the transplant by intensive drugging and irradiation that render the patient thoroughly defenseless against infections. Should the grafting succeed, the guest-marrow-cells show no compunction in setting loose on the host a vicious graft-versus-host-reaction/disease, usually abbreviated as GVHR/GVHD. Transplant means a 'cure rate of perhaps 10%'[275] and 'death for many of the remainder.'[275]

(ix) The lay[14] and learned[271] exhortations to subject more and more ALL cases to the aggressive cure-or-kill therapy rarely amplify the facts[98] that the treatment is merely palliative, increasingly complex, costly in terms of money and therapeutic complications, fraught with uncertainty all the time, an emotional gamble for the patient/relatives/physician, and that regardless of the 'supra-intensive therapy'[274] fatality far exceeds survival.

(x) In 1957, Burkitt discovered in African children a

cancer, called Burkitt's tumour/lymphoma, and now reported from all parts of the world.[22, 266, 276] Burkitt's contribution was held as 'something utterly unique in medical history,'[22] for it pointed to a viral origin of cancer, an assumption that could not[15, 276] be proved right. The initially dramatic way in which Burkitt's tumour responded to chemotherapy led to the hope that this may lead to 'the eventual control of acute leukemia (ALL).'[277]

A parallel may be profitably drawn at this stage between ALL and Burkitt's tumour: Both are essentially made up of 'lymphoblasts,'[98, 276] occur predominantly in children, respond rather dramatically to drugs combined with X-ray therapy, and what is most important, both were and are held as leads towards finding the cause and cure of cancer. Points (i) through (x) and the increasing realization that Burkitt's tumour behaves as obstinately[266] as ALL, put a seal on many a hope best quoted of Burnet:[15] 'To a great many people, medically trained scientists as well as laymen, the pot of gold at the end of the rainbow of medical research is the discovery of the cause and cure of cancer.'

Modus Operandi of Success

A word about the essential mechanism of the success, whatever, against ALL: A patient with a completely blocked esophagus because of cancer would die in a few days – not of cancer, but of starvation, as he would even if the obstruction were by a stricture or a foreign body. Treatment does not tackle the cancer, but the obstruction caused by it, assuring thereby a flow of nutrients, and a lease on life unhampered by the threat of starvation. Similarly, what therapy does in ALL is to remove or minimize in a small percentage of patients, the obstruction/compression of other normal tissues, in the bone marrow, brain and

53

elsewhere, to the point of allowing life to continue, with no change in the basic pathology. It is important to realize that the same cellular force that makes leukemic cells continue multiplying regardless of the therapy also sees to it that normal cells follow suit to populate vital tissues of the body so as to allow the patient to survive and be reckoned as 'cure' or 'remission.' All told, ALL success is an example of palliation – the crowning glory of all forms of cancer therapy.

Yes, It Is Useful to Cure Cancer

'Yes,' said the great Metchnikoff,[99] 'it is useful to prolong human life.' And, despite the blatant iconoclasm of this chapter against cancer therapy, it can be asserted that it is good to cure cancer and thus to prolong useful human life. *Cure* (L. *curatio*, from *cura* meaning care) truly implies *taking care of,* and curing cancer means taking care of a cancer patient, as far as is possible, as best as is possible, and to the maximal well-being of the patient. The physician is undoubtedly the most important intermediary between one's disease and one's dissolution, and the physician's benevolence can mean good life until death. Yes, it is good to cure cancer.

SEVEN

NOT TREATING CANCER

OF all the heresies that have been committed in this book
so far, this may sound as the most unconscionable and
unpardonable. Yet, the weight of the unheard evidence in
favour of this heresy is too compelling to remain unheeded
any longer.

The following case, personally known to the authors, is
illuminating. Mrs. D., a dentist's mother, aged sixty-one
had some vaginal bleeding, for which she was examined
and was found to have carcinoma of the uterus with
metastasis (spread) in the lower vagina. Prior to the
diagnosis – or, rather prior to the treatment – she enjoyed
good health, appetite and sleep, and could move about
freely on her own. The cancer therapist pointed out that
surgery was out of question and recommended that she be
given chemotherapy. The patient pleaded that the disease
did not bother her and that she was not keen on having
anything done to her. The family did not relent and
chemotherapy was started. On the fifth day after chemo-

therapy, she felt very weak, lost her appetite, and had to be hospitalized. The chemotherapy course was duly completed, but the patient never left her bed until her death three months after the treatment, having lost all her appetite, sleep, hair, and her *joie de vivre*, which she had had in full before the treatment. The therapist, who treated Mrs. D. perforce knew that the treatment of choice, *viz.*, surgery, was ill-advised, and he resorted to chemotherapy for treating a known-not-to-respond cancer on the grounds that treatment *must* be given even if there was a snowball's chance in hell that the outcome would be good.

The knowledge of cytokinetics and mode of cancer growth, tells us that Mrs. D surely had had the cancer at least for a decade before there was any discomfort. And even after that, she was at peace with herself and pleaded for being left alone, but in vain. Mrs. D's case illustrates three points: (i) a patient not dis-eased by cancer may be left alone; (ii) the therapy should not be more dis-easing than the patient's dis-ease; and (iii) care should especially be exercised while using cancer chemotherapy. The reason for (iii) should be amply clear from what follows: An eminent authority [100] on cancer chemotherapy has generalized that 'if an agent has certain biological effects, such as carcinogenic, mutagenic, or bone-marrow-depressant activity, it merits testing for chemotherapeutic activity against cancer.' This learned statement ought to convey that all agents presented as anti-cancer were 'carcinogenic' to start with. An editorial [101] titled 'Second neoplasm – a complication of cancer chemotherapy,' annotating an article [102] describing the occurrence of leukemia as a complication of chemotherapy of ovarian cancer, should come as no surprise.

Cancer-realism

Cancer-realism is an imperative for the right not to treat

cancer. The basis for such realism is afforded by the relatively more benign cancers such as chronic myeloid leukemia and chronic lymphocytic leukemia, as well as by the relatively more malignant cancers as of the bronchus, breast, or nasopharynx. An integral part of cancer-realism is Hoerr's law, self-promulgated [278] in 1962: *It is difficult to make the asymptomatic patient feel better*. An obvious corollary to Hoerr's law is that it is very easy to make the asymptomatic patient feel worse, and such a person who is as yet not a patient, is best left untreated, best left unburdened by either diagnostic label or diagnostic procedures.

In 1802, a committee of Scottish physicians wrote a memorandum [103] comprising questions and answers on cancer. This memorandum [103] was first published in 1806, and was reprinted, 'with full justification' in 1967. It may be taken as one of the most cancer-realistic works, published so far, being marked by subtle wit, sound common sense, remarkable dispassion, and brilliant invective. Lamenting the lack of 'an exact definition' of cancer, the memorandum observed: 'It has accordingly happened that a disease, which has been denominated cancer by one medical man, has not been allowed to be such by another; and painful and hazardous operations have been performed by some, which were not thought necessary . . . .' The memorandum also remarked: 'Tumours in the breast, of a considerable size, will often remain in the quiescent state for many years, even to the close of life, if not disturbed by injudicious treatment or extraneous injuries, of which the ancients were well aware. It therefore appears as improper to extirpate these as it does to suffer them to remain, when they begin to be disturbed and can be wholly removed.' The passage of a good 172 years, characterized by unprecedented research-attack against cancer, has not done anything to add a word to, or subtract from, the Scottish wisdom. The above quotes bear thorough relevance even to modern times when (i)

57

many operations are done when unwarranted, (ii) it is possible to live *with* cancer, for many years, and (iii) it is a silent-cancer-turning-symptomatic that calls for treatment.

Ho[104] presenting his experience on 'The Natural History of Nasopharyngeal Carcinoma (NPC), at the Tenth International Cancer Congress 1970, remarked that the duration of the disease – over 97% of the NPC in his series were of the undifferentiated type – varies widely: with no specific treatment, or with radiotherapy, which is only palliative, a patient may live from a few months to over ten years from the time of diagnosis. The patient with the longest survival of thirteen years was an Eurasian, who, all along his 'illness' declined treatment. After thirteen years *with* his cancer, he died at the age of seventy-eight of a heart attack. 'And not so rarely,' we may recall Brooke's words[88], 'cancer itself is overtaken by another disorder and beaten to the final post.'

The chronic leukemias offer frequent examples of cases living for long, when left untreated, or treated only when dis-eased.[105] 'Many of the older patients may die with rather than from the disease.'[51] Asymptomatic patients should *not* be treated, however high the counts and however massive the enlargement of lymph nodes, liver and spleen.[106, 107] Treatment itself may bring in rapid decline by precipitating an acute leukemic crisis.[107] Stevens[108] describes the case of a patient who had lived with her leukemia for the duration of at least seventeen years, and possibly twenty-eight years. She was in good health all along, despite 'extensive infiltration' of the bone marrow by leukemic cells. Asymptomatic, she was trapped into getting her *counts* treated by cancer chemotherapy for the last five years of her life; she then developed varied infections, and eventually succumbed to overwhelming recurrent pneumonia.

Durrant and co-workers[109] reported, in 1971, a 'Comparison of treatment policies in inoperable bronchial (lung) carcinoma'. They randomly allocated 249 patients, with inoperable bronchial carcinoma confined to the chest, to four different groups, each treated differently. One group received no treatment until 'significant' symptoms appeared (the wait-and-see group). The other three groups received treatment whether or not they had symptoms at the time of entry into the trial, and were given radiotherapy, chemotherapy, or a combination of the two. The mean survival in the wait-and-see group was 8.4 months, whereas in the groups treated with radiotherapy, chemotherapy, or their combination, it was 8.3, 8.7 and 8.8 months, respectively. 'The group of patients whose anti-tumour treatment was delayed until symptoms appeared obtained as good palliation as those treated immediately.' The authors[109] of the report felt that their results offered no evidence that immediate treatment by radiotherapy and/or chemotherapy leads to prolongation of survival or to prevention of incapacitating symptoms in patients with inoperable bronchial carcinoma.

The *we-must-operate/treat* therapeutic diehards so insist on the grounds that enough is not known about the untreated diseases. 'On the contrary, if one bothers to scan the literature, there are ample articles on just this subject'[110] showing the 'natural course' of unoperated cholelithiasis,[111], of untreated breast cancer,[112, 113] and so on for gastric-/duodenal ulcer,[114, 115] mitral stenosis[116] and cancers of the esophagus, stomach, colon, rectum, liver, gall bladder, and pancreas.[117]

The Painlessness of Cancer

An important cancerological reality is that all cancers from the time of inception, through five to fifteen years, to the time of diagnosis are 'discreetly hidden'[88] and painless. More importantly, many cancers continue to be painless even after being diagnosed at the primary or the metastatic site. It was the same painlessness of cancer that allowed a Mayo, a Wilkie, or a Dorn to continue to work peacefully up to the time the widespread and inoperable cancer was diagnosed, and death followed fairly soon after the *open and close* procedure. *The Lancet*[118] described oral cancer as an obstinate clinical problem, and lamented that more than half of all patients, in England and Wales with intra-oral cancer, presented themselves at a late stage of the disease. Why at all, one may ask, should such a thing happen when a very small aphthous ulcer in the oral cavity can create hell for a patient through the trigeminal nerve? Why should the oral cancer not imitate the aphthous ulcer? The truth is that it is in the very nature of cancer to be painless during the major part of its existence in the patient's body. Like Nature, cancer is cruel but cancer is kind. And cancer is painless, because it is, teleologically speaking, meant to be so. A patient who 'neglects' a cancer does so because the cancer does not, for long, dis-ease him or her. Which city-dweller 'neglects' a foreign body in the eye or an acute pyogenic abscess in the perianal region?

Not Treating Cancer

Let us now consider the problem of a woman with a silent breast lump: If it is non-cancerous (the chances being more than 2 out of 3),[119] nothing need be done. If it is cancerous, you are too late to do anything. A rational conclusion is that nothing, diagnostic or therapeutic, should be done for this patient. Strange as this proposition may seem, it is fully backed by established cellular and tumoural cancer-realities. An old man found to have a hard but silent prostatic nodule on 'routine checkup' need not be benevolently dragged into the consciousness of having cancer. The diagnosis is, non-committally and correctly, a breast lump, a prostatic nodule, and the like.

It will be a great day for rational medicine when the physician acquires the right not to diagnose, and therefore not to treat, a cancer which is at peace with its owner. Outrageous as this proposition may seem, it pleads that the patient be spared mental death prior to the cancer's turning obtrusive on the patient's senses. It may be argued that unless the patient is warned in advance, he may be caught unawares by the disease. But the warning is unreliable – you tell the patient that he will live 'another three weeks, I won't guarantee you any longer than that!'[9] and he manages to live for many years. The warning is undesirable for it precipitates a sort of posthumous existence with perpetual expectation of the worst, for the patient or even the physician-patient. The warning when expressly denied by the physician, does not spare a patient sudden cancerous or cardiac illness or death. The authors know of a general practitioner's wife, in her forties, declared by some eminent cardiologists of Bombay to be free from any heart problem, dying suddenly of a heart attack barely fifteen days after being given a clean bill of health. This is not an uncommon event, in big cities with big cardiac clinics, where a human being elatedly walks out of the cardiologist's consulting room, with completely normal EKG (ECG), only to collapse to death from a heart attack, barely a few yards away from the clinic.

Cancer, for a long period, exercises discreet silence before dis-easing a person. S. J. Mehta, a staff member of the Tata Memorial Centre, was fit and working before developing symptoms that led to the detection of cancer that had spread to multiple sites without any trace of the primary source.[6] For Sir David Wilkie,[120] 'then, in August 1938, at the age of 56, after a brief spell of declining health . . . . the X-ray confirmation of gastric carcinoma . . . . the end a few days later'. Knowing that the duration of undiagnosable and asymptomatic cancer is pretty long, the cancers in the

61

above two physician-patients must have remained 'discreetly hidden'[88] for many years before turning symptomatic; and for all the time that the cancers were left undiagnosed (and untreated), both the surgeons were mercifully spared the Keatsian 'posthumous existence.'

Physicians, who contemplate the view that cancer may not always be treated would have to bear in mind, however, the modern, litigious society comprising patients prone to turn litigant against the doctors on not getting what they paid for or were ready to pay for. As things stand today, medical, judicial, legal, and general public opinion would tend to hold unimpeachable a 'play-safe' man who treats every cancer case, but would not pardon a doctor refusing to treat until he absolutely must. The position of a such a 'risker' can be rendered progressively safe only by making the physicians and the public – lay, legal, judicial – swallow the insipid but helpful pill that no treatment is also a form of treatment. To help achieve this seemingly impossible aim, enlightened physicians can start an Anoci-Association of Cancer Therapists (AACT) whose motto should be *primun non nocere*. The AACT ought to publicize the unrecognized and unsung benignancy of cancer, the unpredictability of cancer, the hazardous nature of all forms of cancer therapy, the 'damned-if-you-do' and the 'damned-if-you-don't' experience of all cancer therapists, and, above all, that even cancer permits of the patient being left alone. The AACT may eventually manage to get financial aid from government or other agencies by showing that AACT could mean a lot of saving on the enormous monies spent directly or indirectly on cancer every year, the whole world over.

EIGHT

PROGNOSIS IN CANCER

MAKING prognoses is tantamount to prophesying. We do not know how authentic the prophetic role of a doctor is. If the authenticity can be proved, the doctor's right to prognosticate is justified; if not, the physician can be requested to stop playing the prophet. In the widely publicized court trial, [121] the physician's prognosis was that Karen Ann Quinlan, the young American girl in a coma, would die soon if taken off the life-sustaining machines. Her parents pleaded to the court for taking the plugs off so that Karen could die. The court agreed. But Karen did not die. If the physician-prophets could be proved wrong in a case that appeared so clear to most of the people, how could they prove anywhere near right in cancer, surrounded as it is with so much uncertainty, diagnostic and therapeutic?

The State of Prognostic Art

The state of the prognostic art leaves much to be desired. 'Of the trilogy of disease, diagnosis, prognosis, and treatment, prognosis is the most difficult to evaluate. The accurate prediction of things to come is often most baffling, perplexing, and problematic. Caution is essential. The less said the better. Remember that we are endowed with two eyes and two ears but with only one tongue. The implication must be apparent.'[122] This is but natural, for prognosis as a subject has been least touched upon in medical literature. In *A Medical Bibliography* compiled by Morton[123] and published in 1970 in its 3rd Edition, there are 7,534 entries dating back to the time 2250 B.C., of the great Hammurabi; of these, only one entry is on prognosis, *viz. De praesagienda vita et morte aegrotantium* by Prospero Alpino, published in 1601. In *Familiar Medical Quotations*, edited by Strauss[124] and published in 1968, there are more than 7,000 quotations on over 400 subjects – 'from Cathay's Huang Ti, five thousand years ago to present day opinions on transplantation and birth control.' On 'prognosis,' there are eighteen quotes of which only two are from specific works on prognosis; one from Hippocrates' *On the prognostics*, and the other from a small editorial by Robbins,[122] published in 1961 in the *Archives of Internal Medicine*, and quoted from, as above. All told, medical prognostication is more of an art than a science.

Prognosis in Cancer

One who makes a prognosis in cancer, blissfully unaware of his limitations and rather too sure of the ideas of early and late cancer, indulges in two extremes: (1) offering hope when hope may not be rational, or (2) presenting hopelessness when hopelessness may not be warranted. And he can get away with either. The first measure allows him to be condoned on the grounds of his benevolence; the latter measure provides a subtle defence for him, for rarely does a patient surviving longer-than-expected have the heart to find faults with his prognosticator. 'There are doctors who, to show their worth and to be sure of an excuse, make bad seem worse and of the worse make a disaster.'[125]

The reasons why a cancer prognosticator feels so sure of himself are many. His diagnostic and therapeutic skills register *advances* every day. His assessment of a cancer case is seemingly complete – clinical examination, endoscopy, an arsenal of investigations, and the findings at the operation.

Yet, despite this impressive array of aids to prognosis, the prognosticator encounters unreliability, at every stage. What he has always thought to be an early cancer has rarely been so. He takes the small size of a tumour as his guide, but that cannot help him: 'The general assumption that all dwarf-sized cancers must be biologically young is no more valid than the assumption that all human dwarfs must be young because they are small.'[126] The mode of cancer growth renders useless any attempts at detecting the silently growing tumours measuring less than half a centimeter in diameter.

Cancer cytology is highly arbitrary and therefore un-reliable. Histology does not fare any better. 'Contrary to the experience of some workers, we have not found that the histology of biopsy specimens offers any useful guide to prognosis or management.'[104] This 1970 generalization by Ho[104] – in whose series most cancers were undifferentiated – is similar to the 1960 generalization by Sutherland[95] that, at present, prognostically different cancers are often mor-phologically indistinguishable. The grading and staging of cancers represent the valiant efforts by prognosticators at playing the prophet, depending on apparently objective criteria; but 'a given carcinoma may be graded II one day and III the next, or vice versa, depending on the functional tone of the gastrointestinal tract of the pathologist or the barometric pressure.'[127] And what if the grading were to be precise? Writing on the grading of the adenocarcinomas of the colon and rectum, Boyd[128] comments that while statistically it is possible to establish some agreement between the grade, lymph node involvement, prognosis, and so on, 'this does not mean that it is of prognostic value in the individual patient.'

Prognosis in cancer, like in other branches, is a judgement based on circumstantial evidence, but no judgement can be respected when the evidence is largely suspect. To the prognosticator, cancer is what and where he sees it. However, his detecting cancer at one or more sites is no guarantee that the cancer is not additionally present elsewhere. Moreover, what he sees as cancer is an independent, biologically predetermined behavioural entity, that does not permit him to tell: What really is the cancer? Where else is it lurking? What will it do? And when? And when will the patient die of something totally different?

Despite such ignorance, an all too common pitfall is the urge to make favourable prognoses on the basis of 'early' treatment. It was as early as in 1936 that Nathanson and Welch[129] reported that in their series of breast carcinoma, 'patients with the shortest delay of the treatment have the worst prognosis.' Not infrequently, a prognosis of doom proves wrong, and the patient survives, showing that the prognosticator had seen a disaster greater than was in store for the patient.

Role of Statistics

'In individual prognosis,' Hyman[130] remarked, 'statistics function as a weather-vane. From them the practitioner recognizes the wind direction; he knows nothing of wind velocity, or of weather conditions such as temperature, humidity or visibility.' The prognosticating physician is, by and large, unaware of the weather-vane-nature of statistics which come to him as definite, reliable, proved-correct-generation-after-generation figures in authoritative writings on diabetes mellitus,[131] coronary heart disease,[132] hypertension,[133] or various cancers.[20, 134] The prognosticator has nothing to guide him in an individual case – for whom he can, at best, retrognosticate or be wise after the event.

Backed by an implicit faith in the truth of large numbers, the prognosticator finds it convenient to extrapolate the herd data to an individual, ignoring the fact that the extrapolation is fraught with Heisenbergian uncertainty. 'In biological problems, variable factors of considerable complexicity often are present, the necessary consideration of which distinguishes biometry from statistology.'[135] Such warnings escape the eyes of the prognosticator and so he continues to prognosticate despite Heisenberg or Macdonald. Even when he employs statistical prognosis, the prognosticator probably neglects cautionary statements often appearing at the very beginning of the text. 'It is true in diabetes mellitus as in other chronic diseases that the prognosis for the patient is extraordinarily individual.'[131] The cautionary note on an individual is followed by one on a group: 'Generalization with regard to prognosis may be based on averages in special groups and for special complications; nevertheless, wide variations are found in the duration of life and the presence or absence of diabetic sequelae within each group.'[131]

How realistic would it be for the patient were the prognosticator to admit that all that he is offering prophetically is statistical! How unburdening would it be for the prognosticator to realize that, at the level of an individual, he need not prognosticate at all!

The Need for Prognosis

Notwithstanding his crass ignorance on the whether-when-how-and-why of the art, the physician must prog-

nosticate. Brooke,[88] writing on cancer, described prognosticating as 'perhaps the most important act in medicine.' And
perhaps, this is true for altogether different reasons, namely
to share with the patient and his near-ones the usually
unacknowledged medical ignorance on cancer and to let
the patient know that cancer can be as kind as it can be
cruel. Set below are a few suggestions:

1. The time of prognosticating is the time to talk things
over with the patient. It is the time to act as a patient's
friend by providing him with the drive to dare the disease,
and to live with it.

2. Prognosis involves exploring and exposing areas from
where assurance can be had and destroying areas from
where unwarranted fear stems. Cancer patients often live in
depression and it is for the prognosticating physician to pull
them out into living a yea-saying life that meets with the
Kiplingian urge to fill every irretrievable minute with sixty
seconds' worth of distance run.

3. Prognosticating includes protecting the patient against
the tyranny of lay and medical articles rich in well-
intentioned scare-mongering.

4. Prognosticating does *not* include, despite Hippocrates,
guilt-pointing and fault-finding. Carcinoma of the lung in a
smoker, or carcinoma of the stomach in a gourmet, or
carcinoma of the cervix in a woman who has loved life, is no
Dostoevskian story of *Crime and Punishment*. The occurrence
of a lethal laryngeal cancer, in that sage from Dakshine-
shwar, Ramakrishna Paramahansa – whom Wilson[87] calls a
great mystic, a God-intoxicated saint – was certainly no
retribution from a wrathful God.

5. Active Patient-Participation. *What I do not know, is
unfathomable. What I do know, is shareable.* Our 'the-more-we-

know-about-cancer-the-less-we-seem-to-understand-it' pre-dicament has attained sufficient magnitude to enforce the prognosticator to practise the above code of conduct *vis-à-vis* his prognosee.

6. Herd-realism, normal distribution, Gompertz function, curves of disease-specific mortality, etc., are subtle and inexorable indicators of the fact that an individual, despite all his unprecedented, unparalleled and unrepeatable uniqueness, is herd-dependent with respect to many features. In his chapter on the 'Statistical study of tumours', Willis[20] emphasizes that the age distribution of a sufficiently large series of cancer deaths, in a population, provides 'a smooth ideal curve' of normal distribution. This normality of distribution is a herd-function, and, at an individual level, depends on the point of the curve one falls on so as to die of cancer at the age of eighteen, or ninety-eight years. To the person set to die of cancer at eighteen, (as well as to his near ones), it is 'chaotic' that he should be so 'victimized' by Nature. But if he and the others realize that this 'chaos' is a part of the orderly 'ideal' curve, the sense of persecution is likely to be minimized.

7. Prognostication in cancer should include retrognostication consisting in explaining to the patient that his cancer, dis-easing him now, has been with him for five to fifteen years. Further, that the *earliness* or *lateness* of a cancer lies in the mind of the clinician, and not in the cancer.

8. The patient's cancer-realism that he is harbouring a cellular phenomenon of which even the prognosticator is only as wise as he himself can make him an equally important participant in the 'fight' against the disease. In the absence of such realism, the patient suffers from a sense of singular victimization out of the frustration that medicine and medical men are not offering him his due.

9. Prognosticating includes admitting investigational limitations and therapeutic impotence.

10. The cancer-can-be-cured syndrome is no different from the well-recognized ICCU (or ICU) syndrome.[6, 136, 202] (ICCU stands for Intensive Coronary Care Unit. The syndrome is suffered by heart patients admitted to the ICCUs, as also by the medical and paramedical staff attending to them. The ICCU syndrome symbolizes people's and medical men's faith in the marvels of modern medicine bought at an enormous psychic and monetary expense, without good done to anyone.)

The cancer prognosticator must see to it that his patient's body, mind and soul are not additionally burdened with the above syndrome, and that the syndrome does not kill the patient's family while medicine is fruitlessly trying to save the patient.

11. 'Prognosis is a continual process that may extend beyond the patient's death, for the bereaved ones.'[b] This can go a long way towards assuaging the unhappiness, anger and bitterness of the patient's near-ones.[279]

12. An excellent way of winning the confidence of a patient, while prognosticating cancer, is to allude to the not-very-uncommon event of the cancer-patient outliving his cancerologist: Evarts Graham, the famed St. Louis surgeon who introduced 'curative' operation for lung cancer – called 'Graham's operation' – operated on a doctor who survived to see Graham dying of lung cancer 'not diagnosed until it was too late to apply the operation that he had developed.'[280] Such an exercise in medical humility, whereby the healthy-looking physician admits that the diseased prognosee could well outlive him, may find a starting point in an old skip-rope song:

> 'Doctor, doctor, will I die?'
> 'Yes, my child, and so will I.'

70

NINE

IMMUNOLOGICAL ILLUSION

CANCER immunology, also called tumour immunology, is a new and very rapidly expanding[137] science. It is
based on the idea that just as the human body can react
against, and develop immunity to, viruses and bacteria, so
can it react against its own cancer cells to develop immunity
to them. Such immunity is called tumour immunity.
Cancer/tumour immunotherapy is the science of treating
cancer by inducing and/or promoting tumour immunity in
a cancer patient. At present, immunotherapy is given
consideration[138] only if surgery, radiotherapy, and/or
chemotherapy have either failed, or are unlikely to help.

The thrust of cancer/tumour immunological research is
directed to finding out the *foreignness* of cancer cells on the
one hand, and the mechanisms by which the body pre-
sumably develops immunity to them, on the other. The
foreignness of cancer cells supposedly resides in the *antigens*
they carry. The human body's reaction against these *cancer
antigens* resulting in tumour immunity is presumed to be

mediated by the white blood cells—predominantly the lymphocytes.

Today, eulogistic statements[14, 16] on tumour immuno-therapy, on the basis of the 'clear evidence' that medical scientists have, are common. The reality is different. The outcome of the massive research on tumour immunity and immunotherapy has been negative,[5] for the following reasons:

1. Surveying the field of tumour immunology, a science-writer[22] discovered that the science of immunology is so confused—thanks to its Tower of Babel—that one im-munologist cannot make out what the other is talking about.

2. Scientists do not know exactly what *tumour immunity* is. It hasn't yet been defined, and is unlikely to be defined in view of such editorial double-speak: 'This article illustrates that under proper circumstances, tumour immunity can stimu-late tumour growth.'[139]

3. 'Spontaneous tumours,' Willis[20] generalized, 'consisting of a creature's own tissues, rarely if ever act as antigens.' Paraphrased, this means that when not tailored by labora-tory artifacts,[15] a cancer forms an integral part of its owner, and does not exhibit the presumed antigens, nor does the body show any reaction.

4. Point 3 is best illustrated by the fact that in operations on stomach cancer, the stomach wound heals even when the knife has 'actually' run 'through the cancer,'[140] amply proving the integral/non-foreign/self nature of cancer cells, participating as they do in the vital, highly coordinated and complex process of wound healing.

5. Were the body to detect its cancer cells as foreign, it would do so at the very inception of cancer. The fact that

cancer can present itself as a universal and a regular feature, in a predictable proportion of human beings of all ages the world over means that our assumptions about the foreignness of cancer cells are ill-founded.

6. The review of a recent book *Immunotherapy of Cancer in Man: Scientific Basis and Current Status*[141] sums up the situation as one of failure, disappointment, frustration and difficulties, the latest one being that a cancer antigen circulating in the blood may, in fact, protect the cancer against the body's immunological mechanisms.

7. The two arms of tumour immunity are supposed to be (i) the antibodies (humoral immunity), and (ii) the lymphocytes (cellular immunity). The former has long since been recognized as, in fact, protecting a cancer against whatever may be the body's defence.[142] Now, even the cellular immunity is suspect as facilitating the initiation and the growth of a cancer.[143, 144]

8. Even when immunotherapy has succeeded in producing what is termed as tumour immunity, the outcome[144, 145] has not necessarily been beneficial: In some cancer patients, the tumour has regressed somewhat; in others, the tumour has worsened. The reasons for these findings may be clear from the next point.

9. Oettgen and Hellström,[146] writing a chapter in the current Bible, *Cancer Medicine*, raise enough anti-cancer hopes before and after the few lines that follow: 'Thus, it is not simply a matter of deciding whether "immunity" inhibits or fosters cancer. Only if means can be devised to shift the balance between inhibitory and enhancing immunologic forces in either direction can we hope to find a clearer answer.'

10. Point 9 indicates the cancer-promoting danger of immunotherapy. BCG immunotherapy, probably the most

73

talked about, produces 'frequent complications'[143, 147, 148] and presents, in the light of point 9, a cancer-promoting hazard: 'The use of BCG is not without danger since in some circumstances it enhances tumour growth.'[149] In today's world of executives and business management, *The Peter Principle*[150] illustrates how everyone manages to reach his own zenith of incompetence. BCG therapy of cancer, having attained its Peterian zenith of incompetence, is now paving the way for a dubious drug, levamisole,[149] that has proved an 'immunostimulant' with its own unpredictable efficacy and side effects.

The current state of tumour immunity and immuno-therapy has been summed up recently by Hewitt:[137] Genu-ine tumour immunity is probably non-existent because what is *antigenic* in cancer cells is not necessarily immunogenic against those cells. The *in vitro* findings have no counterparts *in vivo*.[98, 281] The 'highly antigenic' animal tumour models bear no relevance to cancer in man.[98, 282] The 'long and inglorious' story of immunotherapy merits only one com-ment − 'a treatment which does not work can hardly be called a therapy.' Hewitt[137] traces the foregoing to the fact that scientists got seduced by, and infatuated with, tumour immunology much before any sound reason was present. The reason is not present even now. All that we have ended up with is, putting immunological interpretations[282] on all obscurities in cancerology.

Regardless, the immunologic show[282, 283] goes on. Re-cently, Mathé and others organized 'The Immuno-can-cerology Week'[283] in Paris, where Feldman of London harped upon the cancerologists' attempts to help mankind immunologically fight its own cancer cells. The meeting concluded that all the research effort of 'immuno-cancerology' was justified.

Let us face it: The science of tumour immunology has one

74

outstanding feature – it has proliferated in a cancerous manner. It is also *fundogenic* – it gets funds for the asking. Yet, when scrutinized scientifically, it reveals itself as a vast exercise of applying utter logic to a false premise – that one's cancer cells aren't part of oneself. No human or animal cancer can be proved foreign (or non-self)[151] to its owner – 'the first warning of the disillusionment to come' having been given to science'way back[3] in 1911. In an individual, the genetic selfsameness of cancer cells (Chapter 2) allows oneself to honour one's own cancer, by declaring it, *à la* Mr. Doolittle in *My Fair Lady*,[152] as 'Me own flesh and blood!'

TEN

CANCER IS UNRESEARCHABLE

BEFORE justifying the heresy that cancer indeed *is* unresearchable, it would be helpful to define research in order to understand science in general, and cancerology in particular.

The dictionary' definition of research has full comprehensiveness, clarity and, in the current context, rich applicability. It defines research as a 'critical and exhaustive investigation or experimentation having for its aim the discovery of new facts and their correct interpretation, the revision of accepted conclusions, theories, or laws in the light of newly discovered facts, or the practical application of such new or revised conclusions, theories or laws.'

Cancerology has *searched* what it could – funds, power, statistics, *but not researched,* as evidenced from its chronic failure to revise its cherished conclusions, much less to put them into practice. The story is singularly one of the denial of seeing the writing on the wall. On science, we might consider what Bobynin says, in Solzhenitsyn's *The First*

Circle:[153] 'What d'you think science is – a magic wand that you just have to wave to get what you want? Supposing the problem's been put in the wrong terms or new factors crop up?' The problem-put-wrong is cancerology's assumption that 'cancer is conquerable.'[14] The new factors that have cropped up are (a) the discovery of the compelling biological features of cancer, and (b) the tell-tale reversals of all therapeutic strategies because of a single unquestionable fact, *viz.*, cancer is a part and parcel of ourselves.

Cancerology has been a professed art of enormous beneficence but with no profound thought or insight. The whole public image of cancerology, Burnet[5] sums up, is one of humanitarianism, but not of biological scholarship. Burnet[15] wonders why so much work for so long by so many top scientists at such a colossal cost has had so insignificant an effect on the prevention or treatment of cancer.

The insurmountable reality about cancer is that it is not amenable to science, being, what Weinberg[154] calls, *trans-science*. All the accessible and analysable facets of cancer – cell, tumour, treatment, cause and prevention, genetics, its very *raison d'être* – for one reason or another, do not lend themselves to prediction by what we know or can do. Set below are the various points/counterpoints *vis-à-vis* each of the above facets.

Cancer Cell

1. Put in Shakespearean style, a cancer cell is, for a person, 'an ill-favoured thing, sir (Mr. Researcher), but mine own.'

2. Not one known structural, biochemical or immunological feature helps in distinguishing a cancer cell from a normal cell.[98, 155, 156, 315]

77

3. A cancer cell suffers from an incurable selfsameness. It, therefore, emerges and multiplies like any other cell, and it falls prey to cytotoxic agents – drugs, X-rays – with no greater willingness than other normal cells of the body. By this one feature of selfsameness, the cancer cell has as it were cured itself, once and for ever, of any selective action by radiotherapy or chemotherapy.

4. A cancer cell carries in itself an indelible stamp of its own uniqueness – rendering itself neither susceptible to a specific drug nor preventable by a vaccine.

5. Cancer cells are, in the human or animal body, in an inexhaustible supply. The reason is simple: recruitment into the cancerous army of many a normal cell that neocancerates[6] to form a cancer cell.

It is little wonder that patients with acute leukemia, even when bombarded with heavy doses of cell poisons over protracted periods, are never free of leukemic cells. This is a classic example of the cancer-realistic fact that whilst some cancer cells can be destroyed, cancer itself cannot.

6. A cancer cell's faculty of leaving its site of origin and migrating elsewhere is predetermined, individualistic, and unpredictable.

7. The uncertainty and individuality surrounding a cancer cell rule out the creation of a cancer-cell-model.

8. Like matter,[157] a cancer cell defies being defined. The best we can do is to paraphrase an academic circumlocution on matter.[158]

> Cancer cell is, what it is
> For it does, what it does.
> And it does, what it does;
> For it is, what it is.

The above lines amplify Smithers'[71] generalization that a

cancer cell is no distinct structural entity, but an organ of behaviour. The same could be said of the overall phenomenon of cancer.

Tumour

The aim of tumour research (clinical cancer research) is, *à la* Kipling, to know the *what, why, when, how, where and who* of tumour formation, in a patient with cancer.

1. A clinician, with all his gadgets, is only wiser after the event. For him to know the *when* of a tumour is impossible whether the patient presents himself for the first time, or after having been treated.

2. The *what* belongs to the realm of individuality of tumours: No two tumours, even in the same person, are exactly alike.[3] All experienced pathologists know that every tumour exhibits its own individuality of microscopic structure.[15, 239]

3. The *why* and *how* belongs to *acausalism*, canceration and tumour-formation being integral parts of life. Much as a 'normal' cell and all its manifestations are a mystery to us, so are a cancer cell and its manifestations.

4. The *what, where* and *who* are predictable certainties at the herd level, but only probabilities at the individual level. The epidemiologic concept of probability can be best amplified by acute lymphoblastic leukemia, a form of blood cancer. Globally, it occurs at the rate of two to three cases per 100,000 population per year with little variation from country to country.[98] Here, the certainty is two to three cases per 100,000 people; who will get it is the quantified uncertainty or probability *viz.*, 1 in 50,000 or 1 in 33,333.

5. The sequence of events from inception of a cancer to tumour formation to dis-ease to death is governed by

79

unpredictability at each step. An earlier event in this sequence is not necessarily followed by the next one. The scare-mongering statistics by cancer societies are generally based on the assumed invariable progression along the above sequence of events. The lack of such inevitable progression, in fact, invalidates the so-called animal-tumour-model used in the laboratory so far.

Treatment

1. The cardinal error of the *cancer-must-be-treated* dogma is the assumption that a patient survives or feels better because of and not despite the treatment. A surgeon[284] who paid a heavy price for such a dogma depicted his experiences in 'A personal account of the after-effects of the modern treatment of carcinoma.' This 1938 article has undiminished relevance in 1978.

2. No mode of cancer therapy can cure cancer; all attack its detectable manifestation.

3. All therapies come on the scene when the silent spread of cancer is a *fait accompli*.

4. Surgery can promote the spread of cancer;[246, 247] most other therapies promote the occurrence of cancer.[6, 8, 15, 101, 102, 248-250]

5. Cancer therapies may ease life, but do not prolong survival, no matter given when and how. To cite some examples: 'In the case of chronic lymphatic leukemia and breast cancer, the mortality rate is independent of the duration of disease. Thus it is reasonable to expect that even a very effective chemotherapeutic agent would not improve the survival of patients with either of these diseases; indeed, it has so far not been possible to demonstrate any effect of chemotherapy on survival. This point was recently re-emphasised for acute myeloblastic leukemia of adults.'[113]

6. The standard 'tumour/test systems' – e.g., Lymphoid leukemia L1210, Sarcoma 180, Adenocarcinoma 755, L5178Y leukemia – are each a borrowed mass of dividing cells, conveniently[6] called *transplanted cancer*. They have nothing to do with human or animal cancers. This dissociation may be realized from the fact that natural or autochthonous cancer is 100% resistant to the drugs that are 100% effective against the so-called transplanted cancer.

7. Cancerology has no cancer-therapy-model bearing relevance to the human or animal situation. Successes gained in test tubes have remained restricted to the test tubes only.

Cause and Prevention

Chapter 4 makes it clear that cancerology has been searching for a cause that never was. What has no cause can have no prevention either.

Genetics

Cancer is an eminent *vertebrate feature* that functions at the herd level, mediated by multifactorial inheritance. The unreasoning dictates of heredity have been epitomized in the Gaiusian dictum – *Damnosa hereditas*. Since cancer has nothing to do with heredity, being basically a herd function that must find expression at some individual level, shall we say, of cancer, that it's an example of *Damnosa herditas*?

It is the corporate gene pool of a herd that determines which type of cancer – nasopharyngeal carcinoma in Chinese populations and leukemia in Jews, around the world – would occur, in which individuals of the herd, and at what different ages. The occurrence of cancer in an individual person is governed not just by his genes but by their corporate interaction with the herd gene pool, a realization that makes cancer not a matter of heredity but *herdity* (herd-ity), and a phenomenon most certainly beyond the ken of genetics – to be candid, *trans-genetics*.

Modern genetics has given up its one-gene-one-character concept, accepting that a single character is controlled by many genes, and *vice versa*. Which of a human cell's 100,000 genes controls the conversion of such a cell into a cancerous one is unknown, more so since the precise definition of a gene itself is unknown.[159] Any attempts at locating cancer gene/s is fraught with problems that are beyond the science of genetics. Burnet[15] has alluded to the current illusion, that *what can happen in* E. coli *can also be made to happen in an elephant*. Cure of cancer through gene-manipulation is as tall an order as that.

Raison d'être of Cancer

The late Leslie Foulds emphasized the need for contemplative research on cancer – to understand it more, than to conquer it. 'Some investigators,' Foulds[3] remarked, 'are fond of saying, "what we need is more facts." The truth is that we already have more "facts" than anybody knows what to do with.' And the incontrovertible facts that we *do* have, are enough to carry us all towards an understanding of cancer.

The approaches that the so-called experimental cancer research has employed lack three essential features – comparability, predictability, and reproducibility. The result, therefore, of all this research has been essentially unhelpful towards the elucidation either of the cause or the cure of cancer. Contemplative cancer research requires three qualities – the humility to consider man on a par with other animals, the comprehensive approach of a generalist and from these two, the acceptance of cancer as a part of living, and dying. Cancer *is* researchable, but only at the level of understanding.

Having understood cancer, what next? Acceptance. To the frontiersmen of science, Ardrey[160] points out, the discovery of natural laws meant no more than that we had come to know certain forces governing the dispositions of man. But for many a 'popular' scientist who came later, such discoveries meant something very different: 'Man could master nature.'

The 'hoi-polloiness' of cancer scientists has been charitably described by Burnet[5] as a beneficent trait, devoid of biological scholarship. The latter quality ought to be evident from the current unwritten law in science-writing and reporting: *Anything that happens to science, happens against cancer.* If a recombinant *E. coli* can be made, cancer can be understood[161]; and when a slime mould shifts from 'amoeba-like feeding to plant-like reproduction,' we are all very near 'a cancer cure.'[162]

ELEVEN

CANCER: A PERSPECTIVE

A S regards cancer, the common man is at the mercy of medical men and the press, both thriving on the paradoxical combination of scare-mongering and cure-prophesying. Needless to say, the various cancer societies represent the best, or even the worst, of the above two forces.

The medical double-speak on cancer is not commonly perceived by the layman. On the one hand, cancer is described as the greatest bugaboo of man,[163] and as a formidable problem almost beyond the comprehension of the human intellect.[164, 165] On the other hand, promises are repeatedly made of the victory against cancer, promises which have reached their climax[166] with the formation of an agency for the outright 'conquest' of cancer. A telling example of medical double-speak may be found in an authenticated, voluminous recent text[167] on cancer: In the preface, the editors pontificate that, 'Several types of human cancer that were hitherto fatal diseases have been cured by drug treatment.' Inside, an authority[168] on drug therapy describes *cure* by drug therapy as 'purely theoretical, since none of the known anticancer drugs has met the conditions for its full realization.'

Due to the persuasive power of the printed word, the press controls lay thinking on cancer. Describing[14, 22, 169] cancer as a totally mysterious, totally inexplicable, and total evil, silent preventable killer is commonplace, occasionally exacerbated by rank paranoia: '. . . a savage cell which somehow . . . corrupts the forces which normally protect the body, invades the well-ordered society of cells surrounding it, colonizes distant areas and, as a finale to its cannibalistic orgy of flesh consuming flesh, commits suicide by destroying its host.'[170]

Having created needless fears over cancer, the press then proposes cures for it too. 'By far the best defense against cancer is an offence.'[14] But what kind of an offence? 'The public has been oversold,' Rutstein lamented:[171] 'Thus, responsible publications cure cancer almost every week.' The pace of cancer research is so great, the press tells us, that by the turn of the century *cancer will be no more*, replacing thus the *Homo sapiens* by the *Homo longevus* enjoying 'life without the prospect of death.'[172] Dawe[18], of the American National Cancer Institute thought that the best analogy of cancer was man himself, proliferating and plundering. Cancer, then, will go; cancerous man will stay for ever!

Who guides the press and how? The scientific community is educating the press, so that the press can guide the public[173]. For example, every year the American Cancer Society sponsors the 'science-writers seminars'. These seminars resemble one very long press conference rather than a serious series of discussions, boosted as they are by lengthy lunches and dinners. 'The Cancer Society apparently believes that there is a connection between a spate of "good-news" cancer stories and the success of its fundraising drive.'[173] The Indian Cancer Society,[169] in a two full-

85

page press release, on February 17, 1978, declared, in the style of the American Cancer Society (see below), cancer as *one of the most curable of all diseases,* only to add that 'work is lagging behind for want of funds.' Individual scientists are not exempt from this ploy. A few years ago, Dr. Robert Good, adorning *Time*[174] magazine's cover, gave a big story inside it, thus testifying to his 'ability to attract research funds and keep his name before the public.'[8]

Greenberg[175] exposed the American Cancer Society's claim about cancer's curability. He[44] quoted Davis, the ACS Science editor: 'Consider the other major death-dealing diseases among which cancer rates second: heart disease, stroke, influenza and pneumonia, diseases of early infancy, diabetes, cirrhosis of the liver, arteriosclerosis, emphysema, nephritis and nephrosis. Cancer is indeed one of the most curable diseases in the country.' Yet, cancer *is* most curable, because all other leading diseases are more incurable than cancer. The medical establishment, indeed, never had it so bad. Despite the 'remarkable technical virtuosity' of modern medicine, it has made hardly any change in the adult life expectancy in the USA, in the last twenty years.[176]

Confusion worse confounded! Such may be the feeling of the reader on perusing the foregoing, and on perceiving that the earlier chapters of this book, and the authors' larger work *The Nature of Cancer,*[6] are uncompromisingly critical of 'almost the whole of contemporary cancer research and cancer treatment.'[177]

A solution to this seeming confusion lies in a perspective on cancer, an understanding of it that stands by us day after day, regardless of the chameleon nature of cancer research and reporting. The understanding of cancer – cancer-realism – apart from offering the delights of studying cancer as an interesting biological phenomenon, can also help towards (i) economizing on cancer, (ii) despecializing

86

cancer, and (iii) accepting cancer as a facet of life in general and a probable part of one's own self, in particular.

Understanding Cancer

A Herd Feature

Cancer is remarkably constant as a herd feature. 'Anybody who spends a little time brooding over the statistics of cancer must be struck by their unexpected constancy. From year to year the figures for each form of cancer show remarkably little variation.' Having so generalized, Glemser[22] cites exact figures: 'Here there are 5,355 cases of cancer of the pancreas one year, 5,427 cases of cancer of the pancreas two years later – almost the same number. Or in another country, there are 218 cases of cancer of the pancreas one year, 221 cases of the pancreas the following year.'

Sir Thomas Browne, the author of *Religio Medici*, compassionately opined that 'the mercy of God hath scattered the great heap of diseases, and not loaded any one country with all.' Cancer occurs everywhere, but in excess nowhere. A high incidence of cancer in one organ in a given country gets balanced by a low incidence of cancer in another organ. Segi and co-workers[178] in their report on mortality due to cancer at selected sites in *24 countries* for the year 1962–63, placed Chile first (among all countries) for carcinoma of the uterus and of the stomach in females, second for carcinoma of stomach in males, twenty-fourth for leukemia in males and twenty-third for the same in females. They[178] placed Israel first for leukemia in males and females, and twenty-fourth for carcinoma uterus. In the *global scatter* of cancer incidence,[179] India shows the highest incidence of cancer of the mouth, pharynx and larynx, but is down below the other countries in the incidence of other cancers.

There are other implications of cancer's constancy as a herd feature. Geographically adjacent countries present startlingly different statistics. Ireland, barely 60 miles away from England, has 10 times more cancer of the lip than England, with reversal of the rates for cancers of lung, breast and uterus. On the other hand, countries poles apart present comparable cancer incidence – lethal prostatic carcinoma shows nearly equal incidence in Canada and New Zealand; women in Scotland and the USA have similar death rates from carcinoma of the colon and the rectum.

A large part of the so-called geographic variations in cancer of different organs is more racial than geographic. For example, as Khanolkar[180] stated: 'Now, what is remarkable from a cancer point of view is that the most common cancer in Hindu women is a uterine cancer. But with the Parsi women the most common cancer is of the breast. . . . Environmentally, their conditions appear to be the same. What is so interesting is that we find some cancers more common in certain groups of people than in other groups living in almost identical circumstances.' While Parsis have a high incidence of breast cancer, they have 'an exceptionally low incidence'[181] of other cancers.

The impartiality with which cancer affects mankind the world over, the constancy of its occurrence at particular sites in a country year after year, its 'startlingly different statistics'[22] for geographically adjacent countries, and equally startlingly similar statistics for countries and people poles apart are *all* indicators of cancer as an integral human/herd feature that has nothing to do with all the postulated cancerogens. The International Agency for Research on Cancer (IARC) Lyon, France, works on and publishes *continental* data on cancer to get clues to the

88

causation of cancer on the basis of 'risk differentials,'[182] which in simple terms means an explanation for the high incidence of oral cancer in India but not in Japan. The IARC fails to mention the reliable-year-after-year data on cancer in a country or in a population, and never refers to the fact that if there are 'high differentials,' there are compensating low or very low differentials, as well.

Summarizing, one could say that cancer is, even at the human level, a discernibly universal feature that is independent of the presumed cancerogens, and is impartial in its global sway. Cancer is a part and parcel of mankind.

At Individual Level: Intrinsic, Time-governed, Senescence

Though you drive Nature out with a pitch-fork, she will find her way back, to triumph in stealth over your foolish contempt.

Horace

Cancer is intrinsic: The intrinsicality of cancer implies that it is the individual's developmental programme that determines whether a cancer would occur. If it is *not* a part of his programme, nothing can cause it; if it *is*, nothing can prevent it.

Cancer springs from one's own flesh and blood. This very fact renders the above Horatian aphorism relevant to human cancer. All therapies put together cannot drive out Nature, manifesting itself as human cancer.

Cancer is time-governed: Man and animals are four-dimensional entities, with time as the fourth dimension. In the words of Portmann,[183] animal life, from its very start as a zygote formed by the union of the sperm and the ovum, is configured time. Put simply, all bodily changes of growth and decay occur along a preset programme, the programme unfolding with the passage of time. It is this time-

89

governedness of cancer which determines the occurrence of an esophageal cancer in a boy aged fourteen years, or a man aged ninety-four years. *The time of such occurrence is normally distributed.*

Portmann,[183] talking of insect metamorphosis, observes that 'the specific formation of the mature organism is prefigured in the egg, though in what way we do not yet know.' Foulds[3] refers to such preprogramming by animal life as a *decision in advance of performance*. Portmann[183] continues: 'We have spoken of the insect, but we are all aware that such temporal processes are embedded in our own life.' Cancer is a temporal process, its programme already embedded in an individual and manifesting itself on the aging of the individual. The preprogramming is once again akin to what Foulds[3] describes as the general phenomena of *decision in advance of performance*, both affirmatively and negatively. The former is exemplified by a puritanical non-smoker ending up with a lung-cancer, and the latter by a chain-smoker smoking his way joyfully into his nineties without any cancer, of the lung or elsewhere.

A corollary of cancer being a part of the temporal unfolding of an individual is that like the unidirectional time-arrow, it is irreversible. No case of cancer, despite widespread folklore, has ever fulfilled the criteria of being labelled as spontaneously regressed or cured. [184, 185.]

Peregrine Laziosi, an Italian monk who lived from 1265 to 1345 A.D., was supposed to have, in his early age, a huge cancerous mass on his leg which disappeared overnight after he desperately prayed to Christ to spare him the amputation. St. Peregrine, O.S.M., the patron saint of cancer patients is often invoked for alleviation and cure of cancer, for which he is best known in Austria, Bavaria, Hungary and Italy.[186]

Can the occurrence of cancer, in an individual, be advanced in time, by making the body age faster? All cytotoxic agents – including X-rays and cancer drugs – are known[187] to accelerate the process of ageing and senescence, thus making a cancer appear earlier. Yet, if cancer is not a part of the individual's programme, such accelerated senescence of an individual means the earlier occurrence of other diseases, *but not cancer*. The much-dreaded X-rays (including those that flow on to female breasts from the widely used mammograph) do not *cause* cancer, but make the cancer appear earlier. In this light, all the so-called cancerogens are 'accelerators of a process that is inherent in the animals',[188] a mechanism discernible from the advancement of the time of cancer occurrence in animals[188] and humans,[189] and best expressed by the title of an article – '*Modus operandi* of carcinogens: Mere temporal advancement.'[190] There is a pithy neologism for cancerogens – they can be called *cancer-preponers*.[6]

Cancer is a form of senescence. 'In fact, death is not natural at all. It's really an avoidable mistake.' Fred Stewart[191] has envisioned the discovery of *The Methuselah Enzyme* that would 'desenesce' the human body and make the afore-quoted anti-death hope a reality. With such an enzyme, the human body just would not senesce. However, Hans Selye,[192] writing in 1965 on 'The Future for Aging Research' as the concluding chapter to *Perspectives in Experimental Gerontology* asserted that 'aging is essentially an ineluctable manifestation' of the entropy that affects both the living and the non-living, and that science does not have *any* evidence to pin its hopes on some 'desenescing' enzyme. If death is inevitable and senescence is ineluctable, then surely there is some basis to link the two: Senescence is the necessary prelude to an intrinsically-timed ontology.

If death is the ultimate function of individual life, death eventuating processes – cancer, vascular diseases – assume a physiologic role. Walter Cannon would have called this the *biolytic/ontolytic wisdom of the body*. Senescence resulting in

91

death is not the outcome of a 'loss of programme,'[193] or a 'meaningless fade-out of genetic programming.'[5] It is an individual-specific, herd-serving, biolytic programme that is, for the individual, no less important nor less purposeful than the biogenic forces that fashion his being and the biotrophic forces that make him grow and exert his ability to survive. 'Why should a purely chemical process in a substance like collagen which has essentially the same composition in all mammals, move faster in some species than in others?. . . Senescence takes a generally similar form in each species, whether judged by the physico-chemical changes in collagen, the incidence of degenerative changes in blood vessels or the high incidence of malignant disease . . . The essence surely is that there is a genetic "programme in time" laid down for each species. There must be a biological clock and a means by which a series of processes can be made to occur earlier or later according to the expediencies of evolutionary survival.'[5] Cancer is but one of a series of senescent forces.

The pantrajectorial occurrence of cancer, from intra-uterine life to old age in man, has prevented it from being called a senescent process, as such a process for reasons etymologic, is expected to occur only in a senile individual. Senescence has been defined as an intrinsic process that increases the probability of the death of an individual.[5, 24, 193] Cancer, at whatever age it occurs, is an intrinsic process that increases the probability of death, whether it be in a child of two years or in a man of eighty years. In fact, its function of heightening the probability of death is more severe when it affects a young individual. In an old person, multiple, mild or moderate senescent processes produce an effectively lethal aggregate. Strehler[193] has put down, as criteria of senescence, intrinsicality, progressiveness and deleteriousness. Now, a child dying of cancer dies of a senescent process. It dies of a process that was intrinsic, deleterious and progressive and which when the child was alive had contributed to the increased probability of death. Nelson's[194] characterization of diabetes mellitus as a disease with wide age range – 'infancy to old age' – during which the disease may manifest itself, should force us to revise our thinking on *senescence:* If cancer and diabetes mellitus in old age are looked upon as senescent manifestations of aging, why should not the same in young age or even in infancy, be considered as anything but forms of senescence?

Summarizing, the hypothesis 'that cancer is an *intrinsic, time-governed, senescent process* is a *gestalt view* on the nature of cancer. The *intrinsicness* does not admit of a cancerogen. The *temporal nature* accounts for the occurrence of cervical cancer in a young girl, and in a woman of seventy years; the *time-governedness* does not permit regression of cancer, a corollary fully substantiated by cancerology; the temporal nature allows the so-called cancerogen to be, more truly, a cancer-preponer. Cancer's senescent nature places it as one of the numerous pre-death forces; the senescent nature excludes cancer as being necessarily a lethal process.

Who Kills Whom?

Foulds[3] has deplored the popular usage of 'military terminology' for cancer, like calling it killer, slayer, enemy and so on. The compelling reason for not calling cancer by such epithets is the confounding fact that, so often, an evident cancer cannot be held responsible for a person's death. Even in the book militarily-entitled *Seeds of Destruction,*[195] the very first chapter speaks of the non-role of cancer: 'Cancers are generally not in themselves fatal; that is, with rare exceptions, they do not produce toxins, or otherwise kill the host directly.'

On the basis of vast survival data of cancers treated and untreated, Waterhouse[196] was inspired to suggest that the diagnosis of cancer should not deprive a person of the benefit of insurance on his life. This accords to cancer an integral part in one's living, without pointing at it the accusatory finger – *You are the killer!*

Patients having cancer, however, *do* die, if not *of,* then *with* their cancer. Many an older individual with chronic leukemia dies *with* the disease.[51] Jones[11] has alluded to the undefined physiological systems that produce death of the patient, and along with him or her, of the cancer. Who kills whom?

Cancer is Trans-scientific

The liver cell is more like a typical cell, with *no* morphological features that make it extraordinary.[197] Yet, it is 'an extremely advanced industrial chemical plant.'[198] The liver cell has been cited here to emphasize the point Smithers[71] made about the cancer cell – both have no definable structural entities, and are only *organs of behaviour.* The cancer cell goes a step further. Liver cells from different animals look and behave similarly; cancer cells don't. Every time a cancer is formed, *speciation* occurs – a new species is formed as it were, unprecedented, unparalleled, unrepeatable. Cancerology's outstanding limitation is its ignorance on its *leitmotif* – the cancer cell.

Weinberg[154] calls a question 'trans-scientific' when it can be asked *of* science, but which cannot be answered *by* science; such a question transcends science. The causality/curability of cancer is one such question. Despite its claims to the contrary, cancerology is a *non-science.*[199]

'A disease is not an entity. ... When the organism is incapable of resistance, as in cancer, *it is being destroyed at a rhythm and in a manner determined by its own properties. . . .* Disease is a personal event. It consists of the individual himself.'[200] This statement by Alexis Carrel adds a further individualistic note to the 'trans-scientific' nature of cancer. Note that Carrel talks of the organism's destruction, but the manner and the rhythm are determined by the organism's own properties. Cancerology thus faces a two-fold unique-ness – of the individual whose biological trajectory is predetermined and unpredictable, and that of the cancer. One more element can be added to this helplessness. Towards studying the causation of cancer, cancerology has never been able to 'cause' a cancer when the cells or the animals had decided otherwise. Whenever it has claimed to 'cause' a cancer, the fallacy has been of *post hoc, ergo propter hoc*.

Given all these crippling limitations, it is easy to under-stand why cancerology has not been and will not be able to do anything against cancer, except studying it as a biophe-nomenon. Here lies the saving grace. Cancer, in many of its facets, is comprehensible, and its behaviour is predictable at a herd level. Science, etymologically means knowing, not doing. Cancer is not trans-science if we aim at understand-ing it. It is so, if we want to manipulate it. More correctly, isn't cancer trans-technique? A part of *Homo sapiens*, but not amenable to the *Homo technicus*! One more, of the Illichian *Limits to Medicine*![201]

Economizing on Cancer

Scientia est potentia; knowledge is power. The knowledge that cancer is essentially non-diagnosable and non-treat-able can, as a concept, propel us towards *not doing* in cancer. Munsif, an eminent Bombay surgeon, was fond of aphorizing that, *a good surgeon is one who knows when not to operate*. What medical man needs to learn, in today's technicalized scene, is when *not* to act. This movement towards *inaction* in medicine is gaining momentum: Malle-son[202] asks: *Need Your Doctor Be So Useless?* Illich diagnoses

Medical Nemesis.[201] Lord Platt's autobiography *Private and Controversial*[203] abounds in 'how to avoid' modern medicine.

Barbara Culliton[204] has recently reported, in *Science,* on the Breast Cancer Detection Demonstration Project conducted jointly by the National Cancer Institute and the American Cancer Society, employing mammography, biopsy and surgery. Pointing out that mammography may diagnose what it had better not, Culliton puts a poser: 'The perplexing question, misdiagnosis aside, is whether surgery and follow-up therapy is really necessary.' To buttress the above, Culliton alludes to a study on prostatic cancer, showing that many a prostatic cancer does not bother its carrier. 'The implication is that one would have done these men no favour by treating them for a disease that was not causing them any problem.' A paragraph from the author's book on cancer,[6] published in 1973, deserves repetition here. 'Doing nothing – neither diagnosing nor treating unless compelled by a cancerous patient's dis-ease – is the highest form of non-empiricism, non-arbitrarism, a kind of *I-respect-you-(the patient)-and-Nature* creed. It is refusing to *interfere,* backing the refusal by a well-deserved assurance or discreet resignation. Agreed that there is *never nothing to be done,*[165] but this "never nothing" should be, whenever warranted, a Jeffersonian "pious" fraud. It cannot be overemphasized that a doctor is an *adviser* first and foremost, a *doer* only when the situation dictates. Should a patient ask him whether the former could be a Ulysses[205] in the world of medical investigations, get killed by chemotherapy, or fall off the Golden Gate Bridge, the doctor's advice should be an assertive "No", for which the patient should neither deny him his fees nor drag him to the court of law.'

The realization that the path of Mary (one of contemplation and inaction) is preferable to that of Martha[206] even in cancerology, can mean a lot of saving on the psychic/

somatic human cost, on animals and as a payoff from these, on the hard cash spent on the overall problem of cancer.

Sparing the Human Psyche

The EKG (ECG) machine, a cardiologist commented, has done more harm than the atom bomb. The harm is in terms of the cardiac neurosis that the machine breeds. Christiaan Barnard [207] talks of the EKG's (ECG) 'electrical squiggle' transforming happy individuals with a purpose in life, into frightened, unhappy creatures of despair.' Harrison [208] remarks that physicians suffer from EKGitis, and Heaven help their patients. Kraus [209] rightly said that 'Diagnosis is one of the commonest diseases.' Marcel Proust [210] lamented that for one disease that doctors cure, they produce a dozen others in healthy individuals by inoculating them with an agent a thousand times more virulent than all the bacteria in the world, *viz.*, 'the idea that one is ill.' Iatrogenic (iatral) diseases, it is commonly believed, [211, 212, 213] can be produced only by treatment. It needs to be appreciated that *diagnosis* itself is an iatrogenic disease.

Diagnostically produced dis-ease is a major problem in cancerology. Despite the fact that the Pap smear, as of today, has doubtful [214] utility towards diagnosing/preventing cervical cancer, the Pap industry flourishes. The terms employed by the cervicologists are indiscreet, to say the least. In a series in which no definite cancer was found, the article had the title 'Positive cancer smear in teenage girls', [215] and carried an exhortation: 'A description of the findings in seventy-seven girls who were less than twenty years of age when they were first discovered to have a positive cancer smear should support the contention that no age limit can be imposed on the application of this cancer screening method: if a girl is old enough to have a vaginal examination she is old enough to have a cervical cytologic examination.' Is this not diagnostic vehemence, diagnostic iatrogenesis? The problem is no different for the breast, as Culliton[204] found (see above). All this diagnosing breeds what King[216] calls *iatrogenic non-disease*, wherein the physician treats his patient for a disease which he has diagnosed but which does not exist. What if it does? We have by now been able to evolve an understanding that if the cancer does not dis-ease, nothing, not even diagnostics need be done, thus saving on all the investigations that otherwise necessarily follow.

Sparing the Human Soma

Having made a diagnosis, treatment is not a must. If the cancer dis-eases, the minimal need be done. Today, mere lumpectomy is followed by results as good as those obtained in breast cancer after radical surgery.[6] Such minimal therapy is applicable to other cancers – prostate,[217] stomach,[140] pancreas[218] and so on.[6]

Cancerologists are not exempt from treating 'people as things,' to earn more money. Over 175 years ago,[103] cancer operations were done more for personal gain than for the patient's benefit; things are not altogether different now.[219] The amount of 'unnecessary surgery'[219] today vindicates Shaw's attack on the 'pecuniary' interests of the surgeons. Surgeon, heal thyself!

Besides the mundane consideration of money, of greater importance is the sheer physical price that the human body must pay every time therapy for cancer is given. 'Doctors', a cancer-patient-turned writer complains, 'play God with my body and life.'[220] Surgery, of necessity, mutilates; chemotherapy and radiotherapy destroy many a normal cell before killing a cancer cell; hormone therapy can mean earlier death from cardiovascular disease;[217] immunotherapy *can* mean the worsening of a cancer. The one dictum that all therapists can safely follow is – *Less is more.*

'Cancer nostrums are big business. They thrive because truly effective drug therapy has not yet been achieved.'[221] When *nothing* really works, everything can be *supposed* or *shown* as working against cancer; and hence the current 'Laetrilomania'. [222] Laetrile, or the anti-cancer vitamin B [17], is condemned as being neither anti-cancer, nor vitaminish, but a money-making fraud, that is at best an expensive and cruel hoax, and at worst dangerous.[220, 223] Laetrilomania is a classic illustration of people's faith that *something* can always be done against cancer. The breeders of this faith are the leaders and the institutes interested in cancer research who, now and again, 'overwhelm the public with electric-guitar-like-clatter in extolling the progress of conventional cancer research.'[222]

Sparing Animals, Cutting Down Research

Not *one* 'cause' of human cancer has been found by animal experimentation,[18] not one cure either.[6, 23] All that the study of cancer in animals teaches us is that the ways of cancer are as 'protean' as the ways of life in all its forms.[224] The SPCA would be fully justified in asking for cutting down of research on animals, on incontrovertible cancerological grounds.

Cancer research is what *anybody does anything* in the sophisticated fields of genetics and molecular biology.[15] An editorial[225] in the BMJ posed a question – 'How relevant is present cancer research?' The editorial asked for an 'agonising appraisal' since it was becoming clear that money spent on cancer was going down the drain. Smithers[71] characterized cancer research as a great field for gathering *bric-à-brac,* one that has lacked not funds but direction. A piece that appeared in *The New York Times,*[226] in a way, typifies cancer research: 'A controversy has arisen over a prominent researcher's purpose in conducting an experiment, in which he induced cancer in a small group of rats. The Federation of American Scientists, a public interest science group, has charged in its monthly newsletter that the scientist conducted the tests merely to make a satiric point. The scientist, Dr. George E. Moore of Denver General Hospital, produced the cancers by inserting sterilized dimes into the peritoneal cavities in the rats' abdomens. Dr. Moore and his collaborator, Dr. William N. Palmer, published their finding in August in a letter headlined, "Money causes cancer: Ban it".'

Cancer research as yet has meant, to use Arley's words,[227] that *more people live on cancer than die of cancer*. What else could it be, given the odd mixture of the Promethean zeal, the cancerophobia, the politicization of cancer. 'I believe, however, that one might justly summarize American medicine as being based on the maxim that what can cure a disease condition in a mouse or a dog can, with the right expenditure of money, effort and intelligence, be applied to human medicine.' What Burnet[228] says about the USA, can be extrapolated to any other country. The Cancer Research Institute in Bombay, founded in 1952, is a grant-in-aid institution, under the Atomic Energy Establishment, Government of India. The five-storey building has most things that a cancer institute would have. In a multi-coloured handout, meant for lay consumption, it gives all adulatory details, including information on the Philips EM 300 electron microscope providing a magnification of up to 200,000 times for the study of normal, pre-cancerous and cancerous tissues. Science is supposed to be the human search for truth. Should not the institute have declared, for once, that like elsewhere in the world, all that the electron microscope has done against cancer is to magnify 200,000 times the human ignorance on cancer?

Fundology of Cancer

The hypothesis is unencumbered by any supporting evidence.
The budget is the only part of the application which seems to
have any substance whatsoever.

Anonymous

The above comment by a member of the National Institute of Health (USA) study section, on an application for funds, exemplifies what Hixson[8] found out about cancerology – *when ignorant of what to do, ask for more funds.* There is the whole science of getting funds:[8, 23, 229] fundology is a good name for it. 'Faculty are immersed in administering the grants acquired, and their prevailing literary exercise is the writing of grant proposals. In short, the academic life has become one not of reflection, but of action.'[230] An unwritten law guiding the above literary exercises is to *ask for more, spend more than you have asked for* and thus assure for yourself a greater and greater grant every 'next year.' In science today, *a man gets known by the funds he begets.*

The annual outlay, in the USA, for cancer research will soon reach the 1 billion dollars mark, and will have to be increased at the rate of at least 100 million dollars a year just to keep pace with inflation.[231] Money is where cancer is. Cancer has pizzazz, luncheons, theatre parties, fund-raising luaus, glamour, and 'in actual dollars and prestige,' even heart/mental disease cannot hold a candle to it[232]. Berman[232] points to the biggest risk in this game – 'what will they do if a cure comes out of it?' They need not worry; cancer will not let them down. Public understanding of cancer may.

There is in the world of cancerology the all too common human failing of keeping up with the Joneses. A linear accelerator acquired by one institution is soon put to shame by a bigger accelerator at another. Berman[232] describes how, when something happens to a bigwig, institutes jump in to make capital out of it. The President of India, Sanjiva Reddy, was discovered to have a lung tumour. With the usual fanfare he was flown to the Mecca of cancer research – the Sloan-Kettering Insitute, New York. Somehow, the Government of India was made to understand that this had to be done, because India didn't have a linear accelerator. India already had one, working. Someone protested, but his voice was drowned in the din of the Establishment. The President's illness is expected to leave the legacy of the prestigious linear accelerator to the major cancer centres in India.

The USA spent 15 billion dollars directly or indirectly on cancer for the year 1968[233]. In 1978 the total bill for health care is expected to exceed 130 billion dollars.[234] Surely, a sizeable part of this must be for the diagnosis, rediagnosis, treatment and retreatment of cancer. Perhaps the USA can afford it. But what of India, Pakistan or Egypt where the majority live below the poverty line? Many an Indian, capable of leading a useful life for himself and his society, goes begging for treatment – be it for tuberculosis, leprosy, chronic poliomyelitis – for want of funds, while cancer research and treatment, with all its sophistries, go on at the major centres in Bombay, Delhi, Calcutta and Madras, where they toe the line drawn by the affluent West. The Indian Cancer Society[169] itself, in its birth, was 'inspired by the monumental service rendered by the American Cancer Society.' No wonder we are out shopping for linear accelerators!

Despecializing Cancer

There prevails in specialized institutes an air of 'we-know-everything-about-the-disease.' Such arrogance is the outcome of a constellation of factors – (i) *after all, specializat-*

ion is the order of the day, (ii) being *specialized,* the institute and its men are most sought after from within and without the country, (iii) the diseasophobia gets tactfully built up by the institute, its peripatetic men, and the affiliated societies, and (iv) the Government's and the public's gullibility is that more funds to a specialized institute makes for more cures.

The outcome of the above specialized-institute-syndrome is twofold: (a) the inevitable 'wiser-than-thou' attitude of the specialists who let the people know their designations and degrees tactfully through the media, and (b) the long waiting lists for an appointment, admission, operation, with the resulting humiliation, sense of despair, anxious-waiting on the part of the patients and their relatives. Our concern here is with the latter point.

With cancer, the most feared name among diseases, it is natural that people seek the speciality centres. Over the years, we have witnessed commendable and voluminous therapeutic work on cancer done by non-specialized 'general' hospitals. The specialized cancer centre in Bombay, The Tata Memorial Hospital does less work on brain cancers than the 'general' hospital (to which the authors are attached) with a neuro-surgery department that has become a referring centre for brain cancer cases, even those from outside Bombay. That is not all. The diagnostic, histopathologic, and autopsic studies on cancer in general hospitals are also significant. What is most important, however, is the fact that a cancer case treated in a general hospital fares no worse than when treated at a specialized centre – a truth that allows global verification. Let us despecialize cancer for the following reasons:

1. Cancer therapy is 'lumpology'. A cancer therapist's chief function is to see a lump, to excise it by surgery and/or reduce its bulk by X-rays, drugs, or hormones.

2. The diagnosis of 'cancer', i.e., the detection of the cancerous lump/s is on the basis of clinical examination and investigations which are not outside the functioning potential of a general hospital.

3. Surgery forms the mainstay of cancer therapy and can be competently performed in most well-equipped general hospitals.

What a cancer patient wants is the necessary 'diagnosis' and 'therapy' without loss of time. Despecializing cancer would help achieve this. How do we despecialize? The answer is simple: Tell the people the truth that it is not important who treats and where, but who and what is treated.

Accepting Cancer

The contemplation of things as they are, without substitution of imposture, without error or confusion, is in itself a nobler thing than a whole harvest of inventions.

Francis Bacon

Bacon's invocation is pertinent, both for the cancer doctor and the cancer patient. The very term *contemplation* carries with it the message of the need for humility, patience, and restraint. To understand cancer is to accept cancer, with grace.

Cancer may easily be accepted as a part of mankind, but what when it comes to one's own self? Somebody has shown the way out.[220] Jory Graham, who has lost both her breasts to cancer that has now spread to her vertebral column and legs, has taken to writing a column inspiringly titled 'A time to live . . .' for the readers of the *Chicago Daily News/Sun-Times*. Like other cancer patients, her first reaction was,

'Why me?' Graham sought the answer in the existentialist creed that the universe as such is absurd and that her cancer is *simply random luck*. The three italicized words would have pleased Blaise Pascal, were he alive today; he would have realized that someone could adopt his *probability child* even when confronted by a personal tragedy. With such an approach, Graham changed her question: 'Why not me?' And with that came a sense of power, a realization that in the time left, 'she can still make choices and decisions.' Graham lives with her cancer, and what is more, she inspires others to do so.

Cancer Can Be Lived With

> *I submit that patients with cancer spend many more patient-years living than dying. There is really much more that could have been said about the patient living with cancer, and dying is certainly not the sole province of the person afflicted with cancer.*

Charles Tashima[285]

A favourite theme of Sir William Osler was to *live in daytight compartments*. He epigraphed one of his addresses with the words of Robert Louis Stevenson:

> *Contend, my soul, for moments and for hours;*
> *Each is with service pregnant, each reclaimed*
> *Is like a kingdom conquered, where to reign.*

Osler did not direct his positivism only to some cancer patients 'for whom time is running out.' He, like Kipling and Stevenson, pleaded that time is running out for everyone afflicted with 'an incurable disease' called 'life.' And since everyone so incurably afflicted with a killer disease – ('The aim of all life is death.')[36] – lives, there is no reason why the presence of another killer disease, e.g., cancer, should mar an individual's zest for living, his *joie de vivre*. The title of Barnard's book *HEART ATTACK—You Don't Have to Die*[207] can be altered and enlarged to read as *CANCER—You Don't Have to Die While You Are Alive.*

Despite affliction with a killer disease, it is possible to live long, be married, remarried, produce children, write medical textbooks, write soul-stirring, Nobel-prize-winning novels, and to make, like Louis Pasteur, epoch-making medical discoveries. And all this despite the inescapable impotence of medicine, so that the foregoing must be taken as evidence of the poorly appreciated *benignancy* of the so-called malignant diseases.

William Boyd,[51] the poet-pathologist, had, in 1948, mucus-cell adenocarcinoma of the parotid. A quarter century has passed and the medical world is still rich with Boyd himself and his books on pathology. His 1970 (eighth) edition of *A Textbook of Pathology*[51] is a book of 1464 pages, 908 illustrations, and has a superb updated text. Alexander Solzhenitsyn had cancer in the mid-1950's from which he recovered. But the cancer has not dried up Solzhenitsyn's pen nor has it deprived him of a marriage thereafter to Natalya from whom he has two sons. And, let us note, all this and a Nobel prize, too, for literature despite a killer disease over a decade ago. 'He has endured,' writes Foote[235] while reviewing Solzhenitsyn's *August 1914,* 'slave camps and near death from cancer. His experiences seem to have produced a strong belief in the existence of an inextinguishable sense of justice in human society and – despite the power and prevalence of evil (and cancer) – a spark of absolute conscience in the individual.'

Sigmund Freud had two killer diseases 'a coronary thrombosis' in his 30's, and an oral carcinoma in his 60's. And yet, these *two enemies within* could not kill Freud who had to be *helped to death by a friend,* his physician/friend Max Schur who twice injected two centigrams of morphine to put him into 'a peaceful sleep,' for ever. In all Freud had 33 operations performed on him for his carcinoma. And yet he *lived* up to the end: 'His ability "to love, to give, to feel, stayed with him to the end," and his creativity endured; in his last years he wrote some of his most significant papers, none of them noticeably influenced by his illness.'[36] This refusal to stunt one's *modus vivendi* was shown equally well by Francis Weld Peabody. Peabody was in 'the last stages of malignant disease' and was taking a round of his ward when, to conserve Peabody's energy, his house officer suggested that he might pass by the next patient, who had a 'typical' pneumonia of the right lower lobe. And the inexhaustible Peabody roared: 'Of course, I shall examine the patient and listen to his chest; although I have auscultated thousands of lungs I have never heard two which sounded alike.'[236] Peabody died in 1927, but in the same year he published an important paper on pernicious anemia in the *American Journal of Pathology*[237]. It was fairly soon after his marriage to Laura that Aldous Huxley developed an eventually fatal carcinoma of the tongue. But the killer disease could not kill the philosopher's *joie de vivre* and he so lived, thought, and wrote that Laura Archers Huxley could write a moving biographical account of her husband, entitled *This Timeless Moment*[37] – a message capable of enlivening every moment of every man.

We have talked so far only of celebrities; we may also draw lessons from the lives of some ordinary men. Sanghavi, the father of a microbiologist and the father-in-law of a consulting physician, of Bombay, was operated upon in May 1967 for a carcinoma of the lower third of the esophagus, which, in the words of Boyd, is 'one of the most hopeless conditions.' With the nodes involved, 'guarded' prognosis was given. In the post-operative period, Sanghavi developed retention of urine from an enlarged prostate for which a prostatectomy was done on him in September, 1967. From that day, till today, when he is seventy-one years old, Sanghavi has not looked back; he eats well, attends to his business, and but for tell-tale operative scars, is as normal as anyone else. The other case is of Dr.

Adenwalla, a general practitioner who was operated upon in 1961 for a colloid carcinoma of the cecum. Following the hemicolectomy, Dr. Adenwalla continued to practise till his death in 1976. In 1971 he was most satisfactorily operated upon for a carcinoma of the large bowel. Yes, it is possible to be struck by a killer disease twice, and yet to be able to refuse to say die.

'The border-line between sympathy and pity is very narrow,' writes Newton-Fenbow,[238] 'and pity is corrosive.' It must be realized that the scare-mongering of modern medicine has created pitiable stigmata out of the so-called killer diseases. Diagnose cancer, coronary heart disease, or hypertension in an individual, and society starts looking at the individual with pity: *Don't do this; don't do that.* 'If one *only* makes a determined effort towards normality when one has to, then one finds (thanks to the pitiers) an increasing number of very valid reasons why today no effort should be made but tomorrow – and when tomorrow arrives one is finally incapable of making any effort'[238]. It is the duty of the physician to spare his patient the burden of paralyzing pity and confusing do's and don'ts from the humans that surround him.

TWELVE

SUMMING UP

'I N my experience, for what it may be worth, it does not usually work out in the long run to be seduced into telling the untruth.' [286] This plea by a cancer doctor can be joined to a declaration made by a cancer patient: 'The time to be honest about cancer is now.' [287] And that has been the aim of the book – to present a *gestalt* view of cancer. Such an approach reveals cancer not as *the villain of the piece* that deserves all the metaphors listed by Susan Sontag [288] but as an interesting, universal fact of biology that also affects humans. This is not easy, given the might and the seeming wisdom of the cancer societies and the cancerologists backed up as they are by senators, lobbyists, 'Benevolent Plotters', engineered columns in the media, and 'the somewhat naive but widely held view that science can make things come out as we would like them to be.' [289]

Facts, however, are on the side of a person wanting to have a realistic approach to cancer. Cancer can be understood – by the lay and the learned – to the point of not fearing its occurrence, and should it occur, towards making the most out of life and getting the best out of medical care. Toward this, we sum up here the epidemiology/cause, diagnosis, prognosis, and the treatment of cancer.

The current epidemic[290, 291] of epidemiologic studies on cancer draws its sustenance from the half-truth that tells you, for example, that cancer of the mouth and throat has a high rate in India, without letting you know that this *highness* gets adequately compensated by low rates of other cancers. This is equally true in Japan or Germany, Tripoli or Timbuktu. In 1926, Cramer[292] pointed out that the apparently greater mortality from stomach and intestinal cancers in Dutch women was compensated by low mortality from cancers of breast and uterus, seemingly higher in English women. We reiterated this in 1973.[6] Burch[293] in 1976, reinforced this to conclude that this global, overall consistency of cancer in its incidence and behaviour reflects an intrinsic human quality, for which no cancerogen need be incriminated. It is time we are cured[6] of cancerogenophobia.[290, 291]

Cancer patients are often overburdened with the guilt that their cancer is the result of some acts of commission and/or omission. This need no longer be. Cancerologists must reassuringly exonerate their patients of any such guilt, in the style of Godwin-Austen,[294] an English consultant neurologist and an authority on Parkinson's disease: 'You must remember first of all,' Godwin-Austen[294] tells his patients in a special booklet, 'that Parkinson's disease has *NOT* resulted from something you have done (or not done) in the past. It is *NOT* caused by overwork or overindulgence, and it is very unusual for Parkinson's disease to be related to injury of any sort.'

What can we say of cancer 'diagnosis' when it is now widely admitted[295, 296] that such a thing is always a late event in the course of the disease! 'Diagnosis,' *is* necessary when a person comes with symptoms. However, the various cancer screening programmes, most vehemently seen with reference to the breast and uterine cervix, seduce into the diagnostic mill a person otherwise completely at peace with herself or himself, and often foist upon the now-patient the diagnosis of cancer or a doubt to that effect. A psychiatrist[297] points out that the very word *cancer* implies, in the mind of the common person, 'pain, disfigurement, hospitalization, debts, inability to care for one's family, dirtiness, loss of sexual attractiveness or function, disability, and possible death,' a complex from which the most highly placed medical[298] men are not exempt. Susan Sontag[288] rightly points out that Karl Menninger has observed (in *The Vital Balance*) that 'the very word "cancer" is said to kill some patients who would not have succumbed (so quickly) to the malignancy from which they suffer.' Not surprisingly, Martin Fischer[81] *proscribed* diagnosis to prevent a 'death sentence' being passed by 'a powerful physician'[299] on a 'powerless patient.'[299]

Comfort[300] has described anxiety-making as a curious preoccupation of the medical profession; unwarranted cancer-diagnosis represents one such preoccupation. The so-called public awareness of breast cancer can mean panicked parents rushing with their frightened daughters to the detection centres, where girls of 8–12 years of age, with asymmetrical growth of otherwise normal breasts, may end up with a permanent loss of breast because of misplaced diagnostic zeal.[301] Screening programmes – described in medical circles[302] as 'succesful business ventures' and as 'frankly commercial' – have proved not only useless but scare-mongering, be it for cancer or coronary artery disease[303, 304] resulting in demands for a decent burial.

The essential non-diagnosability of cancer has foiled the technology and the machines of modern medicine. 'Most of the tools of a doctor used twenty-five years ago fit into a small black bag. Today the typical American physician owns or has access to $250,000 worth of diagnostic equipment . . . . Whenever one tries to link the development of new technology with a coincidental improvement in healing, the answer is always the same. There is none.'[305] This media-assessment is endorsed medically.[306] Prognosis, the other *gnostic* part of clinical cancerology, concerns itself with what a cancer cell or a tumour will do to a patient. The help of technology and machines has also been marshalled toward this, with no gains. Computers have been used to analyse cellular features,[307] only to be plagued[6] by the computer-jargon GIGO – *garbage in, garbage out*. Graham's assertion that 'cancer is inherently unpredictable'[287] is not only so at the gross clinical level as she wants to imply, but at all levels. Regardless, *la technique*[308-312] presses on: the recent report[312, 313] on predicting by 'at least three years' from now the *right* drug for a cancer patient by *pretesting* the drug on the patient's cancer cells grown in a petri dish, is oblivious (a) to the inherently non-specific,[314, 315] toxic,[316] and essentially ineffective[317] nature of 'cancer drug,' (b) to the fact that in a handful[318] of cancers against which the drugs are 'effective', the therapy is attended by unforeseen complications,[98, 316] infections[319] 'and above all frightening uncertainty',[98] (c) to the ability of the one and the same cancer to be made up of more than one cell alone,[6, 20] and finally (d) to the penchant of cancer cells to develop, in no time at all, resistance[274, 320] to a given drug.

While on prognosis, a word or two may be in order on the prognosis of cancer research, itself. Despite such pessimists as Bier[321] – 'all that we know for sure about it can be printed on a calling card,' Burnet,[5, 15] and ourselves,[6] the air is full of tremendous optimism, as may be discerned from Lewis Thomas's latest assertion:[322] 'What is new in medicine is the general awareness that these (senile dementias, arthritis, cancer) are biological problems and that they are ultimately solvable.' Cancerology never had it so good. Greenberg[323] has characterized such proclamations as 'reminiscent of Vietnam optimism prior to the deluge.' Hope, however, springs eternal in the human breast, and cancerologists are no exceptions.

'A common cancer hospital witticism, heard as often from doctors as from patients, is "The treatment is worse than the disease." [288] Why should doctors, of all, let out the truth? They, in fact, do not do so as often and as loudly as they should, but their actions, taken to mitigate their own cancer, betray the truth that they know better the ravages of cancer therapy. Many doctors have 'a strongly pessimistic attitude about treatment of cancer;'[297] no wonder!

A study[324] undertaken to determine to what extent doctors, faced with the prospect of having a cancer, 'practiced what they preached,' revealed some startling facts: Doctors, the 'disappointed' investigators generalized, (a) do not bother to seek an early diagnosis, (b) permit 'unjustifiable delay' before 'curative treatment' is started, and (c) choose as their initial consultant a physician whose culpability for delay is as great as that of a general-practitioner. Doctors, the BMJ[325] recently editorialized, investigate and treat themselves or their relatives inadequately by conventional medical establishment standards. The BMJ asked[326] the Director of Surgery at St. Mary's Hospital, London, what he would do if he had cancer of the rectum. His submission is a revelation by itself: 'I am absolutely certain – and this I am sure will bring the wrath of most colorectal surgeons on my head, but no matter – I would not have an abdominoperineal resection with a colostomy. However managed, however much we delude ourselves, a permanent potentially incontinent abdominal anus is an affront difficult to bear, so that I marvel that we and our patients have put up with it so long. It says much

113

for the social indifference of the one and the social fortitude of the other.'[326]

A la Sontag,[288] doctors invent varied metaphors to demonise cancer and thus justify their 'brutal' therapeutic inflictions on their patients. How do we cure doctors of this dilemma? Erik Erikson[327] in *Hippocrates Revisited* offers some sound advice to doctors in the treatment of their patients: 'What is hateful to yourself, do not do to your fellow men.' It is time that doctors heeded this invocation in full, and in the context of cancer therapy paraphrased it as: *What is hurtful to ourselves, let us not do it to our fellow men called patients.*

Just as 'diagnosis' is imperative, for a person who merits it (see earlier), 'treatment' is necessary for a patient dis-eased by cancer. Jory Graham[287] is quite right in that cancer is more curable than many other diseases. But the cure that Graham refers to has to be understood before it is advertised. 'In 32 years' experience in the U.S.A., Canada, and Great Britain, I have never seen a patient with internal cancer or breast cancer cured in the sense the ordinary man understands the term cure – i.e., to take a disease process away and never have it come back.'[328] Let us accept that every cancer is *curable*, because it is, always, *careable*. And this ability to be cared for includes palliation on the one hand, and life-respecting measures on the other. The venerated cancer bible, titled *Cancer Medicine*[167] reveals its true and glorious purpose when it tells at one place[329] that 'symptomatic treatment' of cancer constitutes the 'best clinical management' and forms 'the backbone of any specific cancer therapy.' Palliation, thus, becomes *the* purpose of cancer therapy. And could one ever talk of radical palliation? It is a sign of coming change, however begrudged,[330] that mutilative cancer therapy is getting replaced by conservative, organ/limb-saving[331] procedures. And this is but a mode of life-respecting. The recent *Hospice Movement*[332, 333] in the West reflects the spreading acceptance of the fact that even a patient with terminal cancer needs, above everything, the dignity of being, both physical and mental.

The oceanic mass of 'facts' on cancer – the outcome of the devoted work of many scientists the world over for so many years – may appear forbiddingly large to permit a useful, practicable synthesis. The concepts and the facts presented in this book speak otherwise – it is possible to integrate the results of clinical and experimental research into a perspectival view appealing and comprehensible to the researchers, doctors, lay people, and above all, the cancer patients. Set below is the gist of the aforemade synthesis.

1. Cancer cannot be caused, cannot be prevented. About its affecting you, adopt therefore a *que sera sera* attitude.

2. Remember that cancer has been with mankind since ages and its occurrence is neither a freak of nor a punishment from Nature. Every cancer is a part of your own self. If you must not love it, you need not hate it either.

3. Each cancer, before it bothers you or your doctor, has been with you for a long time. Early diagnosis/treatment for a cancer is a myth to be buried.

4. For the reasons cited above, it is not at all necessary for you to get yourself screened for cancer. Bother yourself about cancer when, and only when, it really bothers you.

5. Cancer does not always kill nor does it always connote a short post-diagnosis or post-treatment life. Decide to *live* with your cancer until it chooses to die with you.

6. Appreciate that cancer need not necessarily disrupt either your profession or your *joie de vivre*.

7. Since there is nothing like a cure for cancer, insist on being treated symptom-far and no further. Any form of

therapeutic radicalism is despicable overkill by medicine.

8. Must you be treated, seek surgery; should you be irradiated or given chemotherapy, insist on the minimal and be prepared for the cellular levy from head to foot that your body must pay.

9. You owe a duty to your body and soul in the form of a dignified death. Do not deny yourself the dignity of dying.

10. Cancer is a species, class, or ordinal character. You can neither inherit it, nor pass it on to your progeny.

REFERENCES

1. Webster's Third New International Dictionary of the English Language unabridged. Ed. Grove, P. B., G & C. Merriam Co., Springfield, 1971.

2. Virchow, R.: Quoted by Ewing, J., in, Pathological aspects of some problems of experimental cancer research. *J. Cancer Res.*, 1: 71, 1916.

3. Foulds, L.: *Neoplastic Development*. I. Academic Press, London, New York, 1969.

4. Watson, J. D.: Quoted by Greenberg, D. S., in 44.

5. Burnet, M.: *Immunological Surveillance*. Pergamon Press, Oxford, 1970.

6. Kothari, M. L., and Mehta, Lopa A.: *The Nature of Cancer*. Kothari Medical Publications, Bombay, 1973.

7. Love, R.: Obituary – Leslie Foulds. *J. Natl. Cancer Inst.*, 53: III, 1974.

8. Hixson, J.: *The Patchwork Mouse. Politics and Intrigue in the Campaign to Conquer Cancer*. Anchor Press/Doubleday, New York, 1976.

9. Solzhenitsyn, A.: *Cancer Ward*. Bantam Books, New York, 1972.

10. Ingelfinger, F. J.: Cancer! alarm! cancer! *N. Eng. J. Med.*, 293: 1319, 1975.

11. Jones, H. B.: Demographic consideration of the cancer problem. *Tran. N. Y. Acad. Sci.*, 18: 298, 1956.

12. Logan, W. P. D.: Cancer of the breast: no decline in mortality. *WHO Chronicle*, 29: 462, 1975.

13. Dao, T.: Quoted by Greenberg, D. S. in, 44.

14. Brody, J. E., and Holleb, A. I.: *You Can Fight Cancer and Win*. Quadrangle/The New York Times Book Co., New York, 1977.

15. Burnet, M.: *Genes, Dreams and Realities*. MTP, Bucks, 1971.

16. Goodfield, J.: *The Siege of Cancer*. Dell Publishing Co., New York, 1975.

17. Roe, F. J. C.: Cancer as a disease of the whole organism. In, *The Biology of Cancer*. (Ed. Ambrose, E. J., and Roe, F. J. C.) D. Van Nostrand, London, 1966, p.1.

18. Dawe, C. J.: Phylogeny and oncogeny. In, Neoplasms and Related Disorders of Invertebrate and Lower Vertebrate Animals. *Natl. Cancer Inst. Monograph*, 31: 1, 1969.

19. Weiss, P.: Some introductory remarks on the cellular basis of differentiation. *J. Embryol. and Exp. Morphol.*, 1: 181, 1953.

20. Willis, R. A.: *Pathology of Tumours*. Butterworths, London, 1967.

21. Weinstein, I. B.: Genetic code of normal and neoplastic mammalian cells. *Gann Monogr.*, 4: 3, 1968.

22. Glemser, B.: *Man Against Cancer*. Funk & Wagnalls, New York, 1969.

23. Garb, S.: *Cure for Cancer A National Goal*. Springer, New York, 1968.

24. Comfort, A.: *Ageing: The Biology of Senescence*. Routledge and Kegan Paul, London, 1964, p. 57.

25. Knudson, A. G.: *Genetics and Disease*. McGraw-Hill, New York, 1965.

26. Hayflick, L.: The cell biology of human aging. *N. Engl. J. Med.*, 295: 1302, 1976.

27. Griffin, G. E.: World Without Cancer: The Story of Vitamin B$_{17}$. Parts I & II. American Media, California, 1974.

28. Benn, G.: Quoted by Plessner, H.: in, On the relation of time to death. In, *Man and Time: Papers from the Eranos Yearbooks*. Pantheon Books, New York, 1957, p. 249.

29. Zumoff, B., Hart, H., and Hellman, L.: Considerations of mortality in certain chronic diseases. *Ann. Int. Med.*, 64: 595, 1966.

30. Innes, J. R. M.: Malignant disease of domesticated animals. In, *Cancer III*. (Ed. Raven, R. W.), Butterworths, London, 1958, p. 73.

31. Schlumberger, H. G.: Tumours characteristic for certain animal species: A review. *Cancer Res.*, 17: 823, 1957.

32. Dameshek, W., and Gunz, F.: *Leukemia*. Grune and Stratton, New York, 1964.

33. Pickering, G.: Degenerative diseases: Past, present and future. In, *Reflections on Research and the Future of Medicine*. (Ed. Lyght, C. E.), McGraw-Hill, New York, 1967, p. 83.

34. Foote, T.: Books: The taste of hemlock. *Time*, June 12, 1972, p. 62.

35. Haldane, J. B. S.: Cancer's a Funny Thing. *New Statesman*, February 21, 1964.

36. Behavior: Freud and death. *Time*, July 17, 1972, p. 29.

37. Huxley, Laura A.: *This Timeless Moment. A personal view of Aldous Huxley*. Chatto & Windus, London, 1969.

38. *Leukemia Abstracts*. Sponsored by: Lenore Schwartz Leukemia Research Foundation. Prepared by: Research Information Service. The John Crerar Library, Chicago.

39. Gunther, J.: *Death Be Not Proud. A Memoir*. Harper & Row, New York, 1965.

40. Bodley Scott, R.: Cancer chemotherapy – The first twenty-five years. *Brit. Med. J.*, 4: 259, 1970.

41 Lajtha, L. G.: The nature of cancer. In, *What We Know about Cancer*. (Ed. Harris, R. J.), George Allen & Unwin, London, 1970, p. 34.

42. Editorial: 'Early' diagnosis of cancer. *N. Engl. J. Med.*, 275: 673, 1966.

43. Cheatle, G. L.: Important early symptoms in diseases of breast. *Brit. Med. J.*, 2: 47, 1927.

44. Greenberg, D. S.: 'Progress' in cancer research – Don't say it isn't so. *N. Engl. J. Med.*, 292: 707, 1975.

45. Whiteside, M. G., Cauchi, M. V., and Paton, C. M.: Immunotherapy with chemotherapy in the maintenance of remission in acute myeloblastic leukemia. *Med. J.* Aust., 2: 10, 1976.

46. Mathé, G.: Approaches to the immunological treatment of cancer in man. *Brit. Med. J.*, 4: 7, 1969.

47. Wilcox, W. S.: The last surviving cancer cell: The chances of killing it. *Cancer Chemother. Rep.*, 50: 541, 1966.

48. Medicine: What causes cancer? *Newsweek*, January 26, 1976, p. 40.

49. Economy & Business: Reappraising saccharin – and the FDA. *Time*, April 25, 1977, p. 43.

50. Kaplan, H. S.: Discussion on cocarcinogenic substances by

Salaman, M. H. In, *Ciba Foundation Symposium on Carcinogenesis: Mechanisms of Action*. (Ed. Wolstenholme, G. E. W., and O'Connor, M.), Churchill, London, 1959, p. 82.

51. Boyd, W.: *A Textbook of Pathology. Structure and Function in Disease*. Lea and Febiger, Philadelphia, 1970.

52. Coppleson, M., and Reid, B.: *Preclinical Carcinoma of the Cervix Uteri*. Pergamon Press, Oxford, London, 1967.

53. Kessler, I. I.: Husband as agent of cervical cancer. Medical Aspects of Human Sexuality. Aug. 19, 1977, p. 84.

54. Fuller, B. A. G.: *A History of Philosophy*. Oxford & I. B. H. Publishing Co., Calcutta, 1955, part II, p. 152.

55. Kark, W.: *A Synopsis of Cancer*. John Wright, Bristol, 1966, p. 101.

56. Royal College of Physicians of London: *Report on smoking in relation to cancer of the lung and other diseases*. Pitman, London, 1962.

57. Russell, B.: On the notion of cause. In, *Mysticism and Logic*. W. W. Norton & Co., New York, 1929, p. 171.

58. Knebel, F.: Quoted in, *The International Thesaurus of Quotations*. Compiled by Tripp, R. T., Penguin Books, Middlesex, 1976, 975.8.

59. Koestler, A.: The perversity of physics. In, *The Roots of Coincidence*. Vintage Books, New York, 1973, p. 50.

60. Webb, H. E., and Smith, C. E. G.: Viruses in the treatment of cancer. *Lancet*, 1: 1206, 1970.

61. Prehn, R. T.: Immune reaction as a stimulator of tumor growth. *Science*, 176: 170, 1972.

62. Medicine: Mammogram muddle. *Time*, Aug. 2, 1976, p. 45.

63. Fialkow, P. J.: The origin and development of human tumors studied with cell markers. *N. Engl. J. Med.*, 291: 26, 1974.

64. Jelliffe, A. M.: Book review: The Prevention of Cancer. *Proc. Roy. Soc. Med.*, 61: 1072, 1968.

65. Cushing, H.: Quoted in, 124, p. 451.

66. Leading Article: The curability of cancer. *Lancet*, 1: 715, 1954.

67. Park, W. W., and Lees, J. C.: The absolute curability of cancer of the breast. *Surg. Gynec. Obstet.*, 93: 129, 1951.

68. Bloodgood, J. C.: The diagnosis of early breast tumours. *J. Amer. Med. Ass.*, 81: 875, 1923.

69. McKinnon, N. E.: Control of cancer mortality. *Lancet*, 1: 251, 1954.

70. Bunker, J. P., Donahue, V. L., Cole, P., and Notman, M. T.:

Elective hysterectomy: Pro and con. *N. Engl. J. Med.*, 295: 264, 1976.

71. Smithers, D. W.: *On the Nature of Neoplasia in Man*. Livingstone, Edinburgh, London, 1964.

72. Hosokawa, T., Ito., H., Sekina, T., Komuro, N., Tanaka, T., Sekino, S., Miyashita, A., Miura, S., and Ozeki, A.: Studies on the histogenesis of induced chorioepithelioma in rats. *Jikeikai Med. J.*, 23: 85, 1976.

73. Walker, A. E.: Intracranial tumors. In *Cecil-Loeb Texbook of Medicine*, (Ed. Beeson, P. B., and McDermott, W.), W. B. Saunders, Philadelphia, London, 1966, p. 1675.

74. Editorial: Carcinoma of the prostate. *Lancet*, 1: 1259, 1958.

75. Franks, L. M.: The natural history of prostatic cancer. *Lancet*, 2: 1037, 1956.

76. Schiller, W., Daro, A. F., Gollin, H. A., Primiano, N. P.: Small preulcerative invasive carcinoma of the cervix: The spray carcinoma. *Amer. J. Obstet. & Gynec.*, 65: 1088, 1953.

77 Christopherson, W. M., and Parker, J. E.: *Dysplasia, Carcinoma in situ, and Microinvasive Carcinoma of the Cervix Uteri*. (Ed. Gray, L.), C. C. Thomas, Springfield, Illinois, 1964.

78. Siegler, E. E.: Microdiagnosis of carcinoma *in situ* of the uterine cervix. A comparative study of pathologists' diagnoses. *Cancer*, 9: 463, 1956.

79. Way, S.: Methods of discovering carcinoma in situ. Reports of Societies. *J. Obstet. & Gynec. Brit. Emp.*, 67: 150, 1960.

80. Wildavsky, A.: Doing better and feeling worse: The political pathology of health policy. In, *Doing Better and Feeling Worse: Health in the United States*. (Ed. Knowles, J. H.), W. W. Norton & Co., New York, 1977, p. 105.

81. Fischer, M. H.: Quoted in 124, p. 97.

82. Macdonald, I.: The breast. In, *Management of the Patient with Cancer*. (Ed. Nealon, T. F.), W. B. Saunders, Philadelphia, London, 1965, p. 435.

83. Kiricuta, I., and Bucur, M.: Prognostic value of malignant evolutive onset in breast cancer. In, *Oncology 1970, Abstracts*. Year Book Medical Publishers, Chicago, 1970, p. 732, Abstract 1199.

84. Hamblin, T.: Personal view. *Br. Med. J.*, 3: 407, 1974.

85. Billroth, T.: Quoted by Rosemond, G.P., in Newer concepts in the management of patients with breast cancer. *Cancer*, 28: 1372, 1971.

86. Veronesi, U.: Noncurative surgery. In, *Cancer Medicine*. (Ed.

Holland, J. F., and Frei, III, E.), Lea & Febiger, Philadelphia, 1974, p. 530.

87. Wilson, C.: *The Outsider*. Pan Books, London, 1971.

88. Brooke, B. N.: *Understanding Cancer*. Heinemann, London, 1971, p. 105.

89. Watts, A.: Wealth versus money. In, *Project Survival*, Playboy Press, Chicago, Illinois, 1971, p. 165.

90. Stephens, F. O.: 'Crab' care and cancer chemotherapy. *Med. J. Aust.*, 2: 41, 1976.

91. Veronesi, U: Principles of cancer surgery. In, *Cancer Medicine*. (Ed. Holland, J. F. and Frei III, E.), Lea & Febiger, Philadelphia, 1974, p. 521.

92. Weil, R.: Chemotherapy and tumors. *J. Amer. Med. Ass.*, 64: 1283, 1915.

93. Issels, J.: Quoted by Newton-Fenbow, P. in, 238, p. 127.

94. Lewin, I.: Neoplasia. In, *Internal Medicine Based on Mechanisms of Disease*. (Ed. Talso, P. J., and Remenchik, A. P.), C. V. Mosby Co., Saint Louis, 1968, p. 140.

95. Sutherland, R.: *Cancer, The Significance of Delay*. Butterworths, London, 1960.

96. Homburger, F.: *The Biologic Basis of Cancer Management*. Hoeber-Harper, New York, 1957.

97. Lewison, E. F., Montague, A. C. W., and Kuller, L.: Breast cancer treated at the Johns Hopkins Hospital, 1951–1956. *Cancer*, 19: 1359, 1966.

98. Henderson, E. S.: Acute lymphoblastic leukemia. In, *Cancer Medicine*. (Ed. Holland, J. F., and Frei, III, E.), Lea & Febiger, Philadelphia, 1974, p. 1173.

99. Metchnikoff, E.: Quoted by Harrison, R. J., and Montagna, W., in, *Man*. Appleton-Century-Crofts, New York, 1969, p. 337.

100. Karnofsky, D. A.: Experimental cancer chemotherapy. In, *Physiopathology of Cancer*. (Ed. Homburger, F.), Hoeber-Harper, 1959, p. 783.

101. Chabner, B. A.: Second neoplasm – a complication of cancer chemotherapy. *N. Engl. J. Med.*, 297: 213, 1977.

102. Reimer, R. R., Hoover, R., Fraumeni, J. F., Jr., and Young, R.C.: Acute leukemia after alkylating-agent therapy of ovarian cancer. *N. Engl. J. Med.*, 297: 177, 1977.

103. Cancer problems 160 years ago. Institution for investigating the nature of cancer. *Int. J. Cancer*, 2: 281, 1967. This article

originally appeared in the *Edinburgh Medical and Surgical Journal*, 2: 382, 1806.

104. Ho, J. H. C.: Head and neck tumors. The natural history and treatment of nasopharyngeal carcinoma (NPC). In, *Oncology. IV.* (Ed. Clark, R. L., Cumbley, R. W., McCay, J.E ., and Copeland, M. M.), Year Book Medical Publishers, Chicago, 1970, p.1.

105. Green, R. A., and Dixon, H.: Expectancy for life in chronic lymphatic leukemia. *Blood*, 25: 23, 1965.

106. Monti, A.: Diseases of the blood and blood-forming organs. In, *Internal Medicine Based on Mechanisms of Disease*. (Ed. Talso, P. J., and Remenchik, A. P.), C. V. Mosby Co., Saint Louis, 1968, p. 644.

107. Field, J. B., Jr.: Quoted by Green, M. E. in, When to treat leukemia. *N. Engl. J. Med.*, 281, 1018, 1969.

108. Stevens, A. R.: Lymphatic leukemia for perhaps 28 years. *N. Engl. J. Med.*, 281: 448, 1969.

109. Durrant, K. R., Berry, R. J., Ellis, F., Ridehalgh, F. R., Black, J. M., and Hamilton, W. S.: Comparison of treatment policies in inoperable bronchial carcinoma. *Lancet*, 1: 715, 1971.

110. Swan, K. G.: Surgeons and operations. *N. Engl. J. Med.*, 282: 1105, 1970.

111. Wenkart, A., and Robertson, B.: The natural course of gallstone disease. Eleven years' review of 781 non-operated cases. *Gastroenterology*, 50: 376, 1966.

112. Bloom, H. J. G.: Natural history of untreated breast cancer. *Ann. N. Y. Acad. Sci.*, 114: 747, 1964.

113. Zumoff, B., and Hellman, L.: The possibility of predicting the efficacy of cancer chemotherapy in the prolongation of survival. *Lancet*, 1: 878, 1967.

114. Berry, R. E. L.: The surgical and non-surgical treatment of gastric ulcer. *Arch. Surg.*, 79: 326, 1959.

115. Moore, F. D.: The effect of definitive surgery on duodenal ulcer disease: a comparative study of surgical and non-surgical management. *Ann. Surg.*, 132: 652, 1950.

116. Wilson, J. K.: The natural history of mitral stenosis. *Canad. Med. Ass. J.*, 71: 323, 1954.

117. Eisenberg, H.: Trends in survival of digestive system cancer patients in Connecticut, 1935 to 1962. *Gastroenterology*, 53: 528, 1967.

118. Editorial: Oral cancer: A stubborn problem. *Lancet*, 1: 299, 1972.

119. Ratcliff, J. D.: I am Jane's breast. *Reader's Digest* (India),
     September 1972, p. 147.
120. Wilkie, D. P. D.: In, *Great Teachers of Surgery in the Past.* John
     Wright, Bristol, 1969, p. 144.
121. Medicine: A right to die? *Newsweek*, November 3, 1975, p. 42.
122. Robbins, L. L.: Prognosis. *Arch. Int. Med.*, 107: 801, 1961.
123. Morton, L. T.: *A Medical Bibliography.* (Ed. Morton, L. T.),
     André Deutsch, London, 1970.
124. *Familiar Medical Quotations.* (Ed. Strauss, M. B.), Little, Brown &
     Co., Boston, 1968.
125. Anonymous: Quoted in, 124, p. 461.
126. Black, M. M., Opler, S. R., and Speer, F. D.: Structural
     representations of tumor-host relationships in gastric carcinoma.
     Surg. Gynec. Obstet., 102: 599, 1956.
127. Mulligan, R.M.: Introduction to the pathology of cancer. In,
     Management of the Patient with Cancer. (Ed. Nealon, T. F.), W. B.
     Saunders, Philadelphia, 1965, p. 11.
128. Boyd, W.: *Boyd's Pathology for the Surgeon.* (Ed. Anderson, W.),
     W.B. Saunders, Philadelphia, 1967.
129. Nathanson, I T. and Welch, C. E.: Life expectancy and
     incidence of malignant disease: I. Carcinoma of breast. *Amer. J.
     Cancer*, 28: 40, 1936.
130. Hyman, H. T.: Quoted in, 124, p. 461.
131. Krall, L. P.: Clinical evaluation of prognosis. In, *Joslin's Diabetes
     Mellitus.* (Ed. Marble, A., While, P., Bradley, R. F., and Krall,
     L. P.), Lea & Febiger, Philadelphia, 1971, p. 211.
132. Friedberg, C. K.: Angina Pectoris. In, *Cecil-Loeb Textbook of
     Medicine.* (Ed. Beeson, P. B., and McDermott, W.), W. B.
     Saunders, Philadelphia, London, 1966, p. 682.
133. Perera, G. A.: Primary (essential) hypertension. In, *Cecil-Loeb
     Textbook of Medicine.* (Ed. Beeson, P. B., and McDermott, W.),
     W. B. Saunders, Philadelphia, London, 1966, p. 715.
134. Goldberg, I. D., Levin, M. L., Gerhardt, P. R., Handy, V. H.,
     and Cashman, R. E.: The probability of developing cancer. *J.
     Nat. Cancer Inst.*, 17: 155, 1956.
135. Macdonald, I.: The natural history of mammary carcinoma.
     Amer. J. Surg., 111: 435, 1966.
136. Medicine: Who shall die? *Newsweek,* May 24, 1971, p. 52.
137. Hewitt, H. B.: Review of Cancer and the Immune Response by
     Currie, G. A. *Br. Jour. Radiol.*, 48: 516, 1975.
138. Byers, V. S., and Levin, A. S.: Tumor immunology. In, *Basic and*

Clinical Immunology. (Ed. Fudenberg, H. H., Stites, D. P., Caldwell, J. L., and Wells, J. V.), Lange Medical Publications, Los Altos, California, 1976, p. 242.

139. Editorial Comment: The Year Book of Cancer 1973. (Ed. Clark, R. L., and Cumley, R. W.), Year Book Medical Publishers, Chicago, 1973, p. 346.

140. Macdonald, I., and Kotin, P.: Biologic predeterminism in gastric carcinoma as the limiting factor of curability. Surg. Gynecol. Obstet., 98: 148, 1954.

141. McKhann, C. F.: Book review: Immunotherapy of Cancer in Man: Scientific Basis and Current Status. N. Engl. J. Med., 290: 1267, 1974.

142. Roitt, I. M.: Transplantation. In, Essential Immunology. Blackwell, Oxford, 1974, p. 181.

143. Nutting, M. G.: Ascites in malignant melanoma after oral BCG immunotherapy. N. Engl. J. Med., 295: 395, 1976.

144. Saksela, E., and Meyer, B.: Clinical follow-up and the cell-mediated cytotoxicity against HeLa cell in patients with invasive or preinvasive cervical cancer. Med. Biol., 54: 217, 1976.

145. Harris, J. E., and Sinkovics, J. G.: Tumors of man. In, The Immunology of Malignant Disease. C. V. Mosby, Saint Louis, 1970, p. 203.

146. Oettgen, H. F., and Hellström, K. E.: Tumor immunology. In, Cancer Medicine. (Ed. Holland, J. F., and Frei, III, E.), Lea & Febiger, Philadelphia, 1974, p. 951.

147. McKhann, C. F., Hendrickson, C. G., Spitler, L. E., Gunnarsson, A., Banerjee, D., and Nelson, W. R.: Immunotherapy of melanoma with BCG: two fatalities following intralesional injection. Cancer, 35: 514, 1975.

148. Bluming, A. G.: BCG: A note of caution. N. Engl. J. Med., 289: 860, 1973.

149. Wybran, J.: Experimental aspects of immunotherapy. In, Basic and Clinical Immunology. (Ed. Fudenberg, H.H., Stites, D.P., Caldwell, J. L., and Wells, J. V.), Lange Medical Publications, Los Altos, California, 1976, p. 606.

150. Peter, L. J., and Hull, R.: The Peter Principle. Pan Books Ltd., London, 1971.

151. Kothari, M. L., and Mehta, Lopa A.: The nature of immunity. I & II. J. Postgrad. Med., 22: 50, 112, 1976.

152. Lerner, A. J.: My Fair Lady. Adapted from Pygmalion by Shaw, G. B. Penguin Books, Middlesex, 1965.

153. Solzhenitsyn, A.: *The First Circle*. Allied Publishers Pvt. Ltd., Bombay, 1970, p. 88.

154a. Weinberg, A. M.: Science and trans-science. *Minerva*, 10: 209–222, 1972.

154b. Leader: Trans-science. *Med. J. Aust.*, 2: 923, 1975.

155. Homburger, F.: Clinical investigation in cancer research. In, *The Physiopathology of Cancer*. (Ed. Homburger, F.), Hoeber-Harper, New York, 1959, p. 890.

156. Hoch-Ligeti, C.: *Laboratory Aids in Diagnosis of Cancer*. C. C. Thomas, Springfield, Illinois, 1969.

157. Capra, F.: *The Tao of Physics*. Bantam Books, New York, 1977.

158. Ananthachar, V. S.: Do we know what mass is? *Science Reporter*, 6: 287, 1969.

159. Dawkins, R.: *The Selfish Gene*. Oxford Univ. Press, Oxford, 1976, p. 30.

160. Ardrey, R.: *The Social Contract,* Collins, London, 1970, p. 5.

161. Science: DNA research: Not so dangerous after all? *Time*, August 15, 1977, p. 44.

162. Weaver, R. F.: The cancer puzzle. *National Geographic*, 150: 396, 1976.

163. Tainter, M. C.: Medicine's golden age: The triumph of the experimental method. *Tran. N.Y. Acad. Sci.*, 18: 206, 1956.

164. Heiger, I.: Theories of carcinogenesis. In, *Ciba Foundation Symposium on Carcinogenesis: Mechanisms of Action*. (Ed. Wolstenholme, G. E. W., and O'Connor, M.), Churchill, London, 1959, p. 3.

165. Smithers, D. W.: *A Clinical Prospect of the Cancer Problem*. Livingstone, Edinburgh, London, 1960.

166. Page, I. H.: Cancer – conquest or turmoil? *Modern Medicine*, 39: 73, 1971.

167. *Cancer Medicine*. Edited by Holland, J. F., and Frei, III, E. Lea & Febiger, Philadelphia, 1974.

168. Mihich, E.: Pharmacologic principles and the basis for selectivity of drug action. In, *Cancer Medicine*. (Ed. Holland, J. F., and Frei, III, E.) Lea & Febiger, Philadelphia, 1974, p. 650.

169. Indian Cancer Society: Second All India Cancer Convention. *The Indian Express*, Bombay, February 17, 1978.

170. McGrady, P.: Quoted by, Weaver, R. F., in, 162.

171. Rutstein, D. D.: The paradox of modern medicine. In, *The Coming Revolution in Medicine*. Vakils, Feffer and Simons Pvt. Ltd., Bombay, 1967, p.9.

126

172. Kurtzman, J., and Gordon, P.: *No More Dying: The Conquest of Aging and the Extension of Human Life*. Dell Publishing Co., New York, 1977.

173. Culliton, B. J.: Science, society and the press. *N. Engl. J. Med.*, 296: 1450, 1977.

174. Cover Story: Towards cancer control. *Time*, March 19, 1973, p. 30.

175. Greenberg, D. S.: The press and health care. *N. Engl. J. Med.*, 297: 231, 1977.

176. Eisenberg, L.: The search for care. In, *Doing Better and Feeling Worse: Health in the United States*. (Ed. Knowles, J. H.). W. W. Norton, New York, 1977, p. 235.

177. Taylor, D. M.: Book review: The Nature of Cancer. *Brit. J. Radiol.*, 48: 420, 1975.

178. Segi, M., and Kurihara, M.: *Cancer mortality for selected cancer sites in 24 countries*, No.4 (1962–1963), Sendai (Japan) Tohoko University School of Medicine, Dept. of Public Health, Japan, 1966.

179. Dunham, L. J., and Bailer, J. C.: World maps on cancer mortality rates and frequency ratios. *J. Nat. Cancer Inst.*, 41: 155, 1968.

180. Khanolkar, V. R.: Quoted by Glesmer in 22, p. 122.

181. Moore, D. H., Sarkar, N. H., Kramarsky, B., Lasfargues, E. Y., and Charney, J.: Some aspects for the search for a human mammary tumor virus. *Cancer*, 28: 1415, 1971.

182. Higginson, J.: Foreword. In, *Cancer Incidence in Five Continents*. Volume III – 1976. International Agency for Research on Cancer, Lyon, 1976, p. vii.

183. Portmann, A.: Time in the life of the organism. In, *Man and Time*. Pantheon Books, New York, 1957, p. 308.

184. Everson, T. C., and Cole, W. H.: *Spontaneous Regression of Cancer*. W. B. Saunders, Philadelphia, 1966.

185. Comments: Spontaneous regression of primary cutaneous melanoma. *Med. J. Aust.*, 2: 759, 1975.

186. Pack, G. T.: St. Peregrine, O.S.M. The patron saint of cancer patients. *Ca*, 17: 183, 1967.

187. Curtis, H. J.: Biological mechanisms of delayed radiation damage in mammals. In, *Current Topics in Radiation Research*. (Ed. Ebert, M., and Howard, A.), North-Holland Publishing Co., Amsterdam, 1967, p. 139.

188. Shimkin, M. B.: Pulmonary tumors in experimental animals. *Adv. Cancer Res.*, 3: 223, 1955.

189. Bizzozero, O. J., Johnson, K. G., and Cicocco, A.: Radiation-related leukemia in Hiroshima and Nagasaki, 1946–1964, *N. Eng. J. Med.*, 274: 1095, 1966.

190. Kothari, M. L., and Mehta, Lopa A.: *Modus operandi* of carcinogens: Mere temporal advancement. *J. Postgrad. Med.*, 15: 101, 1969.

191. Stewart, F.M.: *The Methuselah Enzyme*. Bantam Books, New York, 1972.

192. Selye, H.: The future for aging research. In *Perspectives in Experimental Gerontology*. (Ed. Shock, N. W.), C. C. Thomas, Springfield, Illinois, 1966, p. 375.

193. Strehler, B. L.: *Time, Cells and Aging*. Academic Press, New York, London, 1968.

194. Nelson, W. E.: Diabetes mellitus. In, *Textbook of Pediatrics*. (Ed. Nelson, W. E.), W. B. Saunders, Philadelphia, 1969, p. 1155.

195. Maugh II, T. H. and Marx, J. L.: Seeds of Destruction. *The Science Report on Cancer Research*. Plenum Press, New York, 1975.

196. Waterhouse, J. A. H.: *Cancer Handbook of Epidemiology and Prognosis*. Churchill, Livingstone, London, 1974.

197. Loewy, A. G., and Siekevitz, P.: *Cell Structure and Function*. Amerind Publishing Co., New Delhi, 1974, p. 7.

198. Nilsson, L., and Lindberg, J.: *Behold Man*, Harrap, London, 1973, p. 143.

199. Kothari, M. L., and Mehta, Lopa A.: Cancerology – Science or Non-Science. *Journal of Postgraduate Medicine*, 24: 68, 1978. be published).

200. Carrel, A.: *Man, the Unknown*. Macffaden Publications, New York, 1961, p. 162.

201. Illich, I.: *Limits to Medicine. Medical Nemesis: The Expropriation of Health*. Marion Boyars Publishers Ltd., 1976.

202. Malleson, A.: *Need Your Doctor Be So Useless?* George Allen & Unwin, London, 1973.

203. Platt, R.: *Private and Controversial*. Cassell. London, 1972.

204. Culliton, B. J.: Mammography controversy: NIH's entrée into evaluating technology. How important is early detection? *Science*, 198: 171, 1977.

205. Rang. M.: The Ulysses syndrome. *Canad. Med. Ass. J.*, 106: 122, 1972.

206. Huxley, A.: *The Perennial Philosophy*. Fontana Books, Collins, 1966, p. 299.
207. Barnard, C.: *Heart Attack. You don't Have to Die*. W. H. Allen, London, New York, 1972, p. 78.
208. Harrison, T. R.: In retrospect: some pride and more folly. *Am. J. Med. Sci.,* 269: 111, 1975.
209. Krauss, K.: Quoted in, 124, p. 97.
210. Proust, M.: Quoted in 124, p. 472.
211. D'Arcy, P. F., and Griffin, J. P.: *Iatrogenic Diseases*. Oxford Univ. Press, London, 1972.
212. *Diseases of Medical Progress*. Edited by Moser, R. H., C. C. Thomas, Springfield, Illinois, 1964.
213. Pyke, D. A.: Iatrogenic disease. In, *The Fontana Dictionary of Modern Thought*. (Ed. Bullock, A., and Stallybrass, O.), Fontana/Collins, London, 1977, p. 296.
214. Knowles, J. H.: The responsibility of the individual. In, *Doing Better and Feeling Worse: Health in the United States*. (Ed. Knowles, J. H.), W. W. Norton, New York, 1977, p. 57.
215. Ferguson, J. H.: Positive cancer smears in teenage girls. *J. Amer. Med. Ass.,* 178: 365, 1961.
216. King, L. S.: Editorial: Let this be a lesson to you! *J. Amer. Med. Ass.,* 219: 81, 1972.
217. Bailar, J. C. III.: Estrogen therapy for prostatic cancer. In, *Progress in Clinical Cancer*. IV. (Ed. Ariel, I. M.), Grune and Stratton, New York, 1970, p. 387.
218. Crile, G., Jr.: The advantage of bypass operations over radical pancreatoduodenectomy in the treatment of pancreatic carcinoma. *Surg. Gynec. Obstet.,* 130: 1049, 1970.
219. Duval, M. K.: The provider, the government, and the consumer. In, *Doing Better and Feeling Worse: Health in the United States*. (Ed. Knowles, J. H.), W. W. Norton, New York, 1977, p. 185.
220. Medicine: A time to write. *Time,* November 14, 1977, p. 40.
221. Gellhorn, A.: Clinical cancer chemotherapy. In, *Physiopathology of Cancer*. (Ed. Homburger, F.), Hoeber-Harper, 1959, p. 1013.
222. Ingelfinger, F. J.: Editorial: Laetrilomania. *N. Eng. J. Med.,* 296: 1167, 1977.
223. Martin D. S.: Laetrile – a dangerous drug. *Ca,* 27: 301, 1977.
224. Dawe, C. J.: Comparative neoplasia. In, *Cancer Medicine*. (Ed. Holland, J. F., and Frei, III, E.), Lea & Febiger, Philadelphia, 1974, p. 193.

225. Leading Article: How relevant is present cancer research? *Brit. Med. J.*, 3: 45, 1969.

226. Altman, L. K.: Cancer experiment spurs controversy: New York Times, 23rd October 1977, p. 27. Quoted in *Current Contents*, 21: 12, 1978.

227. Arley, N.: Applications of stochastic models for the analysis of the mechanism of carcinogenesis. In, *Stochastic Models in Medicine and Biology*. (Ed. Gurland, J.), The Univ. Wisconsin Press, Madison, 1964, p. 3.

228. Burnet, M.: Concepts of autoimmune disease and their implications for therapy. In, *Reflections on Research and the Future of Medicine*. (Ed. Lyght, C. E.), McGraw Hill, New York, 1967, p. 9.

229. Mirkin, H. R.: *The Complete Fund Raising Guide*. Public Service Materials Center, 1973.

230. Susser, M.: *Causal Thinking in the Health Sciences. Concepts and Strategies of Epidemiology*. Oxford Univ. Press, New York, 1973.

231. Fredrickson, D. S.: Health and the search for new knowledge. In, *Doing Better and Feeling Worse: Health in the United States*. (Ed. Knowles, J. H.), W. W. Norton, New York, 1977, p. 159.

232. Berman, E.: *The Solid Gold Stethoscope*. Macmillan, New York, 1976, p. 169.

233. Higginson, J.: Overall anti-cancer strategy. In, *Cancer-Painstaking Progress*. Documenta Geigy, Ciba-Geigy Ltd., Basle, 1971.

234. Thomas, L.: On the science and technology of medicine. In, *Doing Better and Feeling Worse: Health in the United States*. (Ed. Knowles, J. H.). W. W. Morton, New York, 1977, p. 35.

235. Foote, T.: Books: Witness to yesterday. *Time,* September 25, 1972, p. 52.

236. Peabody, F. W.: Quoted in 124, p. 164.

237. Peabody, F. W.: The pathology of the bone marrow in pernicious anemia. *Amer. J. Path.*, 3: 179, 1927.

238. Newton-Fenbow, P.: *A Time to Heal. A Personal Testimony of Dr. Issels' Cancer Treatment*. P. Souvenir Press, London, 1971.

239. Spriggs, A. I., Boddington, M. M., and Halley, W.: Uniqueness of malignant tumours. *Lancet,* 1: 211, 1967.

240. Scheinfeld, A.: *You and Heredity*. (Ed. Haldane, J. B. S.), Chatto and Windus, London, 1939.

241. Roberts, J. A. F.: *An Introduction to Medical Genetics*. Oxford Univ. Press, London, 1970.

242. Higginson, J., and Muir, C. S.: The role of epidemiology in elucidating the importance of environmental factors in human cancer. *Cancer Detection and Prevention*, 1: 79, 1976.

243. Schneiderman, M. A.: Eighty percent of cancer is related to the environment. *Laryngoscope*, 88: 559, 1978.

244. Staszewski, J., Slomska, J., Muir, C. S., and Jain, D. K.: Sources of demographic data on migrant groups for epidemiological studies of chronic diseases. *J. Chron. Dis.*, 23: 351, 1970.

245. Haenszel, W., and Kurihara, M.: Studies of Japanese migrants. I. Mortality from cancer and other diseases among Japanese in the United States. *J. Nat. Cancer Inst.*, 40: 43, 1968.

246. Willis, R. A.: *The Spread of Tumours in the Human Body*. Butterworths, London, 1952.

247. Lewis, M. R., and Cole, W. H.: Experimental increase of lung metastases after operative trauma (amputation of limb with tumour). *Arch. Surg.*, 77: 621, 1958.

248. Windeyer, B.: Applications of radiobiology to radiotherapy. In, *Modern Trends in Radiotherapy*-2. (Ed. Deeley, T. J.), Butterworths, London, 1972, p. 1.

249. Kligerman, M. M.: Principles of radiation therapy. In, *Cancer Medicine*. (Ed. Holland, J. F., and Frei, III, E.), Lea & Febiger, Philadelphia, 1974, p. 541.

250. Copeland, M. M.: The biologic aspects of cancer of the breast: A challenge. *Amer. Geriatrics Soc.*, 36: 97, 1978.

251. Gunz, F. W.: Chronic lymphocytic leukemia. In, *Cancer Medicine*. (Ed. Holland, J. F., and Frei, III, E.), Lea & Febiger, Philadelphia, 1974, p. 1256.

252. Lo Buglio, A. F.: Leukemic reticuloendotheliosis: A defined syndrome of an ill defined cell. *N. Eng. J. Med.*, 295: 219, 1976.

253. *Cell Differentiation: A Ciba Foundation Symposium*. Edited by De Reuck, A. V. S., and Knight, J. Churchill, London, 1967.

254. DeRobertis, E. D. P., Saez, F. A., and De Robertis, Jr. E. M. F.: Cell differentiation and cellular interaction. In, *Cell Biology*. W. B. Saunders, Philadelphia, 1975, p. 441.

255. Bhatnagar, S. M., Kothari, M. L., and Mehta, Lopa A.: *Essentials of Human Embryology*. Kothari Medical Publishing House, Bombay, 1977, p. 54.

256. Daver, A., and Agerup, B.: β_2-Microglobulin and cancerembryonic antigen in intestinal cancer. *Danish Med. Bull.*, 25: 91, 1978.

257. Shields, R.: Ectopic hormone production by tumours. *Nature*, 272: 494, 1978.

258. Ellison, R. R.: Acute myelocytic leukemia. In, *Cancer Medicine*. (Ed. Holland, J. F., and Frei, III, E.), Lea & Febiger, Philadelphia, 1974, p. 1199.

259. Gius, J. A.: Palliative treatment of cancer. In, *Fundamentals of General Surgery*. Oxford & IBH Publ. Co., Calcutta, 1965, p. 241.

260. Gius, J. A.: Cancer and cacotelic operations. *Surg. Gynec. & Obst.*, 108: 743, 1959.

261. Moertel, C. G.: The esophagus. In, *Cancer Medicine*. (Ed. Holland, J. F. and Frei, III, E.), Lea & Febiger, Philadelphia, 1974, p. 1519.

262. Feinstein, A. R.: Symptoms as an index of biologic behaviour and prognosis in human cancer. *Nature*, 209: 241, 1966.

263. Cowdry, E. V.: *Etiology and Prevention of Cancer in Man*. Appleton-Century-Crofts, New York, 1968.

264. Nelson, J. H., Jr.: Uterine cervix. In, *Cancer Medicine*. (Ed. Holland, J. F., and Frei, III, E.), Lea & Febiger, Philadelphia, 1974, p. 1733.

265. Colebatch, J. H.: Developing role of anticancer drugs in cancer treatment. *Med. J. Aust.*, 1: 265, 1978.

266. Leading Article: Non-endemic Burkitt's lymphoma. *Brit. Med. J.*, 1: 1508, 1978.

267. Leading Article: The price of survival in childhood leukemia. *Brit. Med. J.*, 1: 321, 1978.

268. MRC's Working Party on Leukaemia in Childhood: Testicular disease in acute lymphoblastic leukaemia in childhood. *Brit. Med. J.*, 1: 334, 1978.

269. Baumer, J. H., and Mott, M. G.: Sex and prognosis in childhood acute lymphoblastic leukaemia. *Lancet*, 2: 128, 1978.

270. Editorial: Testicular infiltrates in childhood leukaemia: Harbour or harbinger. *Lancet*, 2: 136, 1978.

271. Jacobs, P.: Editorial: The curing of human leukaemia – Fact or fancy? *S.A. Medical Journal*, 53: 610, 1978.

272. Thomas, E. D., Buckner, C. D., Fefer, A., Sanders, J. E., and Storb, R.: Efforts to prevent recurrence of leukemia in marrow graft recipients. *Transplantation Proceedings*, 10: 163, 1978.

273. Gale, R. P. for the UCLA Bone Marrow Transplant Team: Approaches to leukemic relapse following bone marrow transplantation. *Transplantation Proceedings*, 10: 167, 1978.

274. Santos, G. W.: Bone marrow transplantation in acute leukemia – remaining problems. *Transplantation Proceedings*, 10: 173, 1978.

275. Editorial: Bone-marrow transplantation. *Lancet*, 1: 859, 1978.

276. Ziegler, J. L.: Burkitt's tumour. In, *Cancer Medicine*. (Ed. Holland, J. F., and Frei, III, E.), Lea & Febiger, Philadelphia, 1974, p. 1321.

277. Burchenal, J. H.: Geographic chemotherapy – Burkitt's tumour as a stalking horse for leukemia. Presidential Address to a meeting of the American Association for Cancer Research in Denver, Colorado, May 1966.

278. Hoerr, S. O.: Hoerr's law. *Amer. J. Surg.*, 103: 411, 1962.

279. Wessel, M. A.: Care of the cancer patient. *N. Eng. J. Med.*, 295: 1435, 1976.

280. Nealon, T. F., Jr.: Cancer: Some personal reflections and an overview. In, *Management of the patient with cancer*. (Ed. Nealon, T. F., Jr.), W. B. Saunders, Philadelphia, 1965, p. 3.

281. Prager, M. D.: Specific cancer immunotherapy. *Cancer Immunol. Immunother.*, 3: 157, 1978.

282a. International Conference on Immunobiology of Cancer. Edited by Friedman, H., and Southam, C. *Ann. N.Y. Acad. Sci.*, Vol. 276, 1976.

282b. Carter, S. K.: Immunotherapy of cancer in man: Current status and prospectus. *Ann. N.Y. Acad. Sci.*, 277: 722, 1976.

283. The Immuno-cancerology Week in Paris. *La Medicine En France*, 26: 13, August 1978.

284. Furnivall, P.: A personal account of the after-effects of the modern treatment of carcinoma. *Brit. Med. J.*, 1: 450, 1938.

285. Tashima, C. K.: Care of the cancer patient. *N. Eng. J. Med.*, 295: 1435, 1976.

286. Jones, H. W.: Comment on Should the doctor tell the patient that the disease is cancer? by Gilbertsen, V. A., and Wangensteen, O. H. *Ca*, 12: 82, 1962.

287. Graham, J.: A time to live: biweekly column in *Chicago Daily News* and now in *Chicago Sun-Times* since July 9, 1977.

288. Sontag, S.: 1. Illness as metaphor. 2. Images of illness. 3. Diseases as political metaphor. *New York Review of Books*, Jan. 26, Feb. 9, Feb. 23, 1978.

289. Marston, R. Q.: Cancer research in the US. *Nature*, 273: 321, 1978.

290. Werner, E. R.: Cancer epidemic? A symposium on carcinogens. *Bull. N. Y. Acad. Med.*, 54: 347, 1978.

291. Curnen, M. G. M.: Epidemiological outlook on cancer. *Bull. N.Y. Acad. Med.*, 54: 349, 1978.

292. Cramer, W.: The new outlook on cancer. *Brit. Med. Jour.*, 1: 175, 1926.

293. Burch, P. R. J.: *The Biology of Cancer: A New Approach.* MTP, England, 1976.

294. Godwin-Austen, R. B.: *Parkinson's Disease – A booklet for patients and their families.* Parkinson's Disease Society, U.K., 1977, p. 1.

295. Handley, R. S.: Conservative surgery for breast cancer. *Jour. Royal Soc. Med.*, 71: 246, 1978.

296. Malpas, J. S., and Whitehouse, J. M. A.: Medical management of malignant disease. In, *Progress in Clinical Medicine*, Churchill, Livingstone, London, 1978, p. 236.

297. Holland, J.: Psychologic aspects of cancer. In, *Cancer Medicine*. (Ed. Holland, J. F., and Frei, III, E.), Lea & Febiger, Philadelphia, 1974, p. 991.

298. Ellis, H.: If my wife had cancer of the breast. *Brit. Med. J.*, 1: 896, 1978.

299. Hellegers, A. E.: Biologic origins of bioethical problems. In, *Obstetrics and Gynecology Annual.* Vol. 6, 1977. (Ed. Wynn, R. M.), Appleton-Century-Crofts, New York, 1977, p. 1.

300. Comfort, A.: *The Anxiety Makers*, Panther Books, London, 1968.

301. Leading Article: Breast lumps in adolescent girls. *Lancet*, 1: 260, 1978.

302. Knox, E. G.: Multiphasic screening. *Lancet*, 2: 1434, 1974.

303. Editorial: Multiphasic screening in general practice. *Lancet*, 1: 29, 1978.

304. Bate, J. G.: Cervical cytology. In, *Contemporary Obstetrics and Gynaecology*. (Ed. Chamberlain, G. V. P.), Northwood Publ., London, 1977, p. 341.

305. Knaus, W.: Modern hospital becomes a warehouse for machines. Reprinted from *Washington Post* in *Indian Express*, Aug. 4, 1978.

306. Round the World: United States: Health care – where the money goes. *Lancet*, 1: 926, 1978.

307. Wied, G. L., Bahr, G. F., Bartels, H., and Bibbo, M.: Cancer cell identification by computer (Program TICAS). Tenth International Cancer Congress. Abstracts. Houston, Texas, U.S.A., 1970, (*Abstract* 908), p. 561.

308. Muhm, J. R., Brown L. R., and Crowe, J. K.: Use of computed

tomography in the detection of pulmonary nodules. *Mayo Clin. Proc.*, 52: 345, 1977.

309. Burwood, R. J.: Ultrasound in malignant disease of the abdomen: a review. *Jour. Royal Soc. Med.*, 71: 199, 1978.

310. Juret, P., Delozier, T., Mandard, A. M., Couette, J. E., Leplat, G., and Vernhes, J. C.: Sex of first child as a prognostic factor in breast cancer. *Lancet*, 1: 415, 1978.

311. Ritman, E. L., Robb, R. A., Johnson, S. A., Chevalier, P. A., Gilbert, B. K., Greenleaf, J. F., Sturm, R. E., and Wood, E. H.: Quantitative imaging of the structure and function of the heart, lungs, and circulation. *Mayo Clin, Proc.*, 53: 3, 1978.

312. Salmon, S. E., Hamburger, A. W., Soehnlen, B., Durie, B. G. M., Alberts, D. S., and Moon, T. E.: Quantitation of differential sensitivity of human-tumor stem cells to anticancer drugs. *N. Eng. J. Med.*, 298: 1321, 1978.

313. Medicine: The petri dish and the patient: Predicting which drugs will work on cancer patients. *Time*, June 26, 1978, p. 55.

314. Stock, J. A.: The chemotherapy of cancer. In, *The Biology of Cancer*. (Ed. Ambrose, E. J., and Roe, F. J. C.), D. Van Nostrand Comp., London, 1966, p. 176.

315. Clarkson, B. D.: Current concepts of leukemia and results of recent treatment programs. *Transplantation Proceedings*, 10: 157, 1978.

316. Hersh, E. M.: Modification of host defense mechanisms. In, *Cancer Medicine*. (Ed. Holland, J. F., and Frei, III, E.), Lea & Febiger, Philadelphia, 1974, p. 681.

317. Editorial: Human tumours in mice and rats. *Lancet*, 1: 138, 1978.

318. Zubrod, C. G.: Introduction. In, *Cancer Medicine*. (Ed. Holland, J. F., and Frei, III, E.), Lea & Febiger, Philadelphia, 1974, p. 601.

319. Bodey, G. P.: Infections in patients with cancer. In, *Cancer Medicine*. (Ed. Holland, J. F., and Frei, III, E.), Lea & Febiger, Philadelphia, 1974, p. 1135.

320. Wheeler, G. P.: Alkylating agents. In, *Cancer Medicine*. (Ed. Holland, J. F., and Frei, III, E.), Lea & Febiger, Philadelphia, 1974, p. 791.

321. Bier, A.: Quoted in *Familiar Medical Quotations*. Ed. Strauss, M. B.), Little, Brown & Co., Boston, 1968, p. 476.

322. Thomas, L.: Biostatistics in medicine. *Science*, 198: 675, 1977.

323. Greenberg, D.: The war on cancer: Official fiction and harsh facts. *Science and Governmental Report*, Vol. 4, December 1, 1974.

324. Robbins, G. F., Macdonald, M. C., and Pack, G. T.: Delay in the diagnosis and treatment of physicians with cancer. *Cancer*, 6: 624, 1953.

325. Leading Article: If I had. *Brit. Med. J.*, 1: 874, 1978.

326. Dudley, H. A. F.: If I had carcinoma of the middle third of the rectum. *Brit. Med. J.*, 1: 1035, 1978.

327. Erikson, E. H.: The golden rule and the cycle of life. In, *Hippocrates Revisited*. (Ed. Bulger, R. J.), Medcom, New York, 1973, p. 181.

328. Riggall, F.: Treatment of Cancer. *Brit. Med. J.*, 1: 1029, 1952.

329. Selawry, O. S., and Hansen, H. H.: Lung cancer. In, *Cancer Medicine*. (Ed. Holland, J. F., and Frei, III, E.), Lea & Febiger, Philadelphia, 1974, p. 1473.

330. Block, J. B.: Drugs for cancer. In, *Drugs of Choice 1978–1979*. (Ed. Modell, W.), C. V. Mosby, St. Louis, 1978, p. 580.

331. Editorial: Osteosarcoma: Advances in treatment or changing natural history? *Lancet*, 2: 82, 1978.

332. Editorial: Hospice care. *Lancet*, 1: 1193, 1978.

333. Medicine: A better way of dying. *Time*, June 5, 1978, p. 55.

GLOSSARY

Terms have been defined with reference to medicine in general and cancer in particular. An attempt has been made to go beyond the mere dictionary meaning so as to provide a wider perspective. Related words are mentioned in parenthesis at the end of the explanation.

Adenocarcinoma.   Cancer arising in a gland.

Allogeneic.   Originating in a genetically different individual, but from the same species.

Analgesic.   Pain-relieving drug, such as aspirin.

Anoci-Association.   An association based on the Hippocratic motto *primum non nocere*, meaning that the least that a therapy should do to a patient, is to do no harm.

Antigen.   A substance, that on introduction into the body, excites a highly specific response in the form of antibody (a protein) and/or cells (lymphocytes). An antigen's specific reactivity with antibody/cells allows laboratory detection of its presence in blood or a tissue. Some cancers carry on their cells and/or secrete into the blood antigens, of which the carcinoembryonic antigen (CEA) is an example. CEA, found most commonly with cancer of the gastrointestinal tract, is detected in the laboratory by demonstrating its reactivity with a specific antibody.

Aphthous ulcer.   Small, painful ulcer/s accompanying inflammation of the mouth.

Arteriosclerosis.   Thickening and hardening of arteries, a common accompaniment of ageing.

Autochthonous.   Arising from an individual's own tissues; not transplanted.

Benign.   Not threatening health or life; opposite of malignant; non-cancerous. A benign tumour/lump has microscopic features resembling a normal tissue.

Bronchial cancer.   A bronchus is a subdivision of the air-passages beyond the trachea (windpipe). Cancer of the lung usually starts in a large bronchus, and thus is often referred to as bronchial cancer or bronchial carcinoma.

Burkitt's tumour.   A lymphoma with characteristic microscopic picture, commoner at younger age. Also called *Burkitt's lymphoma.*

Cancerability.   It is the faculty of a normal cell to *cancerate* and thus turn into a cancer cell.

Cancerogen.   A substance supposedly producing cancer. Also called, *carcinogen.* A substance that assists a *cancerogen* is called *cocancerogen,* and one that opposes its action is called *anticancerogen.* Similarly, *cocarcinogen* and *anticarcinogen.*

Cancerogenesis.   The production of cancer. Also called *carcinogenesis.*

Cancerologist.   A cancer specialist. Also called *oncologist.* The speciality is called *cancerology* or *oncology.*

Cancerotrophic.   An agent promoting the growth of a cancer.

Cancer-realism.   An approach to cancer based on cancerologic, cytologic and biologic facts. Such facts constitute *cancer-realities.*

Celluloma.   A lump or a mass made up of cells. *-oma* as a suffix indicates swelling; hence, lipoma, fibroma, astrocytoma, melanoma, etc.

Chemotherapy.   Therapy by drugs.

Cholelithiasis.   Formation of stones in the biliary tract. Gall stones.

Choriocarcinoma, gestational.   A cancer arising from the chorionic covering of a foetus, and growing in the uterus of the mother.

Chronic.   Any illness characterized by long duration, or frequent recurrence over a long time, and often by slowly progressing severity; opposite of acute.

Chronic lymphocytic leukemia.   Often abbreviated as CLL. A type of slowly growing leukemia characterized by the excessive proliferation of lymphocytes all over. A disease mainly of the middle and old age.

Chronic myeloid leukemia.   Often abbreviated as CML. A type of slowly progressing leukemia, characterized by the excessive proliferation of granular white blood cells, starting in the bone marrow and then appearing in the blood and elsewhere. A disease mainly of the middle and old age.

Cirrhosis.   A chronic disease characterised by progressive destruction and hardening of the liver.

Collagen.   The fibrous protein that provides the scaffold for the animal body, being one of the principal skeletal substances binding cells and tissues together.

Colposcopy.   Examination of the vagina and cervix with an instrument called colposcope that provides illumination and magnification.

Cytodifferentiation.   The process whereby a cell changes its character to turn into another type of cell. Also called *differentiation.*

Cytokinetic.   Related to the process of cell division and proliferation, the science of which is called *cytokinetics.*

Cytologist.   One specializing in the study of cells. (Cytology).

Cytotoxic.   Toxic or lethal to cells. X-rays and 'anticancer' drugs are cytotoxic agents, being indiscriminately toxic to both normal and cancerous cells.

Desenesce.   Rejuvenate.

Diabetes mellitus.   What is commonly known as diabetes is medically termed as diabetes mellitus (sweet diabetes) because of the patient passing sugar in the urine. Such diabetes is to be distinguished from diabetes insipidus, wherein the patient passes large quantities of 'insipid' urine.

Disease.   The term is derived from old French *desaise* (*des* – absence of, and *aise* – ease), and really means dis-ease or lack of ease. The etymologic emphasis has been lost in medical science so that the word disease is freely used even though the so-called disease – a cancerous mass in the prostate or the breast – in no way dis-eases the owner.

Dysplasia.   Literally, abnormality of a tissue. In current fashion, it implies cellular abnormalities of the lining epithelium of the cervix of the uterus, that 'a pathologist recognizes as abnormal, yet not to a degree he is willing to call cancer.'

E. coli.   Short form for Escherichia coli, a bacterium normally found in billions in the human and animal intestine.

Ectopic. Out of the normal place. A hormone is normally secreted by its special gland. When it is also secreted elsewhere by another tissue, it is called ectopic hormone.

EKGitis. A term to describe the inordinate faith of the doctor or the patient in the diagnostic and prognostic usefulness of the electrocardiogram (ECG), sometimes abbreviated as EKG.

Follow-up. The medical practice of periodically reassessing and recording the condition of a patient following diagnosis and/or treatment.

Gaussian distribution. A theoretical frequency distribution that is bell-shaped, symmetrical and of infinite extent. Also called *normal distribution.* Many a biologic feature, related to health or disease, exhibits gaussian distribution.

Gerontology. Science of ageing, and of the problems of the aged.

Grading. A mode of describing the severity of a cancer by grading it as Grade 1 through 4. The severity of a cancer is assumed to be directly proportional to the departure of its cells from normality, when seen through a microscope. A cancer belongs to Grade 1 when most of its cells are near-normal in appearance and arrangement, and to Grade 4 when most cells look abnormal in appearance and arrangement.

Histological. Related to the study of tissue – normal or cancerous – with a microscope. (Histology, Histologist).

Hodgkin's disease. A form of lymphoma with special microscopic features.

Hysterectomy. Surgical removal of the uterus.

Iatrogenic. Produced by a doctor. Also called *iatral.*

Immunological. Related to the science of immunology that studies the nature of antigen/antibody reactions and cells that possibly mediate the immunity (defence mechanisms) of the body against a disease. (Tumour immunity/immunology, Immunotherapy).

Intercurrent disease. The occurrence of an unrelated disease in a cancer patient.

Leukemia. Cancer of the white blood cells.

Linear accelerator. Specialized machine for X-ray treatment of cancer. Such a machine, by the tremendous acceleration it imparts to electrons, produces high energy X-ray beams, that allow a patient to be treated 'in one or two minutes.'

Lumpolytic.   An agent that causes dissolution, albeit temporary, of a cancerous lump.

Lymphoma.   Cancer arising in lymphoid tissues. Unlike in leukemias, the involvement of the bone marrow by the cancerous cells, and their presence in the blood stream are uncommon.

Malignancy.   In cancerology, used as a synonym for cancer; hence, malignant tumour or malignant lesion. In medicine in general, malignant implies grave severity of a disease; thus, malignant fever, malignant hypertension, malignant malaria. A malignant tumour shows miscroscopic features supposedly characteristic of cancer. Opposite of benign.

Mammography.   Study of the breast by X-rays.

Melanoma.   A skin cancer arising from its pigmented cells; can also arise from the eye, mucous membrane, and other tissues.

Metastasis.   Spread or transfer of disease (cancer, infection) from its site of origin to another site not directly connected with it. (Metastatic, Metastasize).

Multifactorial inheritance.   See *Polygenic inheritance.*

Mitral stenosis.   Narrowing of the mitral valve of the heart.

Nasopharyngeal carcinoma.   Cancer of the nasopharynx, the region of the throat behind the cavity of the nose.

Nephritis.   Inflammation of the kidney.

Nephrosis.   Non-inflammatory, degenerative disorder of the kidney.

Neoplastic development.   Development of cancer. *Neoplasm*, literally meaning new(ly formed) tissue usually connotes cancer, although such process also occurs in inflammation, wound healing, etc.

Ontolysis.   Dissolution of one's own self.

Palliative.   Any therapeutic measure that affords relief, but no freedom from the disease. (Palliation, Palliatable).

Pernicious anaemia.   A form of anaemia which, before the discovery of its therapy with vitamin B_{12}, was inexorably fatal.

Polygenic inheritance.   The occurrence of cancer in an individual is governed by many unidentifiable genes (hence called polygenic/multifactorial inheritance) which, in coordination with the genes of the entire herd, determine whether or not cancer would occur. And such genetic governance in an individual is quantitative and not qualitative. All humans *can* develop cancer; only *some* do, for in them the quantitative gene effect is sufficient enough to carry them beyond a certain genetic threshold.

Polygenic inheritance has been invoked to explain the occurrence of a wide variety of diseases ranging from congenital malformations like cleft palate to common diseases like peptic ulcer, heart attack, diabetes, or hypertension.

Primary.   In cancerology, it refers to the site where the cancer first originates; hence, primary site, primary cancer, primary growth, and so on. When a cancer, taking off from the primary site, establishes itself at other additional site/s physically discontinuous from the primary, it is said to have formed secondary or metastatic cancer. From the secondary site, the whole process of metastasis can be repeated.

Probability.   Etymologically and simply, it means likelihood. Epistemologically, it implies a state of knowledge that is less than certainty but greater than ignorance. Epidemiologically, it means certainty at the herd level which, being numerically smaller than the number forming the herd, must of necessity be a matter of chance, likelihood or probability when expressed at an individual level. Such measurement or quantitation of uncertainty is called probability.

The epidemiologic concept of probability can be best amplified by acute lymphoblastic leukemia, a form of blood cancer. Globally, it occurs at the rate of 2 to 3 cases per 100,000 population per year with little variation from country to country. Here, the certainty is 2 to 3 cases per 100,000 people; who will get it is the quantified uncertainty or probability viz., 1 in 50,000 or 1 in 33,333.

Prognosis.   The act or art of foretelling the course of a disease; also, it means the prospect of survival and recovery from a disease.

Prophylactic.   A preventive or protective measure against a disease. (Prophylaxis).

Radical therapy.   Drastic and supposedly thorough treatment for a cancer. Usually applied to surgery, but also to other modes of therapy and to therapeutic combinations. *Supraradical therapy* represents the extreme of therapeutic radicalism.

Radiotherapy.   Treatment of cancer (or any other disease) by X-rays.

Recombinant E. coli.   A type of bacterium with a new combination of DNA assembled in the laboratory through the recently developed technics of genetic engineering.

Recruitment.   When a normal cell cancerates to join the already existing cancer, it is called recruitment or neocanceration.

142

Remission. A temporary abatement of the symptoms of a disease.

Sarcoma. Cancer arising in the connective tissue – especially bone, cartilage, muscle, and fascia. Sarcoma differs from carcinoma in that the latter arises from the cells lining the skin and internal organs, or the cells forming glands such as the liver, thyroid, pituitary, etc. The term cancer encompasses both carcinoma and sarcoma, and is freely used, e.g., bone cancer, breast cancer, stomach cancer, and so on.

Senesce. Grow old; wither.

Smegma. The cheesy, sebaceous matter that collects between the glans penis and foreskin in a male, or around the clitoris and labia minora in a female.

Spontaneous. Not induced, as by a 'cancerogen.'

Stage. Staging is the clinical practice of assessing and expressing the evolution and the spread of cancer in a patient. Stages are expressed in numbers and/or letters, e.g., O, I, II, III, IV for cervical or vaginal cancer, or O, A, B_1, B_2, C, D_1, D_2 for bladder cancer. Stage O indicates minimal cancer; IV/D_2 indicates most advanced cancer. Staging is to be distinguished from grading, a judgement passed on the microscopic features of a cancer.

Stricture. Abnormal narrowing of the lumen of a tubular organ (gullet, intestine, windpipe), by various causes such as inflammation, cancer, etc.

Syndrome. A set of symptoms and signs that occur together in disease; a symptom complex.

Thanatologists. Specialists in *thanatology,* the science of death and dying.

Thermography. The technique of converting the temperature pattern in an organ into a photographic image, as an aid to diagnosis.

Thrombophlebitis, migrating. Also called *thrombophlebitis migrans.* It means the occurrence of inflammation and thrombosis of veins at multiple sites and of a shifting nature; occurs uncommonly in cancers as of the stomach or pancreas.

Trigeminal nerve. The nerve carrying sensations from the head and face region, and innervating muscles of mastication.

Tumour. A lump, swelling, or a protuberance. Often used as connotative with cancer.

Tumour systems.   Cells from a cancer that arose once upon a time in an animal are cultured over the years, by being serially bred in test tubes and animals. Such cells when inoculated in specially prepared animals form masses that are called *transplanted cancer*. Such 'cancers' constitute tumour systems against which drugs are tested.

Xerography.   Also called *xeroradiography*. Study of breast by obtaining its image by a technique similar to that operating in a *XEROX* machine.

INDEX OF NAMES

(Including Bibliography)

The names and the references cited in the text have been indexed, each followed by the reference number in parenthesis, and/or the page/s on which it appears.

147

INDEX OF SUBJECTS

Burkitt's tumour/lymphoma, 46, 53, 138

Cancer
  age incidence, 21
  age-specific mortality rate, 21
  aggravation of, 44
  and biologic trajectory, 29
  antigens, 71, 73
  as a biological phenomenon, 16, 95, 112
  as careable disease, 114
  as class character, 116
  as curable disease, 114
  as disease of whole organism, 36
  as herd feature, 87–89
  as human problem, 24–30
  as integral part of self, 77, 115
  as intrinsic process, 34, 89, 93
  as killer disease, 41
  as ordinal character, 116
  as racial feature, 20
  as senescent process, 21, 91, 93
  as solution, 23
  as species character, 116
  as systemic disease, 46
  as time-governed process, 89–90, 93
  as vertebrate feature, 81
  as universal phenomenon, 16, 89, 89
  at individual level, 89
  benign lumps diagnosed as, 38
  causa sine qua non of, 13, 33
  causeless, 31–35
  causes of death in, 22
  cell, 71, 77–79, 94, 112, 138
    an organ of behaviour, 79, 94
    and normal cell, 16–18
    biochemical features, 77
    definition of, 40, 41
    foreignness of, 71, 73
    genetic content of, 17
    immunological features, 77
    integral/non-foreign/self nature of, 72
    last surviving, 30

  proliferation, 25
  self-determined rhythm of, 18
  selfsameness of, 75, 78
  size, 21, 25
  structural features, 77
  compatible with long life, 24
  course of, 18
  cytologists, 40
  definition of, 11, 57, 78
    biological, 12
  demonized, 114
  diathesis for, 44
  field of origin, 28
  gene/s, 82
  highly palliatable, 43
  histological variety, 29
  histologist/s, 40
  immunology, 71–75
    disillusionment with, 75
    fundogenic, 75
    research, 71, 72
  immunotherapy, 71
  in animals, 99
  in Canada, 88
  in children, 21
  in Chile, 87
  in chimney-sweeps, 31
  in England, 88
  in herd, 19, 20–21
  in Hindu women, 88
  in inbred animals, 19
  in India, 87
  in individual, 18–20
  in Ireland, 88
  in Israel, 87
  in migrants, 20
  in New Zealand, 88
  in Parsi women, 88
  in rats, 100
  in Scotland, 88
  in USA, 88
  incidence, world over, 87
  incurable, 48
  inherent nature of, 21
  invasiveness of, 21
  link with life, 35

152

153

154

155